How the Brain Works

HOW
THE BRAIN
WORKS

A New Understanding of Human

Learning, Emotion, and Thinking

——— ———

LESLIE A. HART

——— ———

Basic Books, Inc., Publishers

NEW YORK

Library of Congress Cataloging in Publication Data

Hart, Leslie A.
  How the brain works.

  Includes bibliographical references and index.
  1. Brain. I. Title.
QP376.H29   612'.82   74-79275
ISBN 0-465-03102-1

Printed in the United States of America
DESIGNED BY VINCENT TORRE
75 76 77 78 79   10 9 8 7 6 5 4 3 2 1

To my wife, Jane

and with a pat on the head to the memory
of the best of all possible standard poodles,
our Bobo, who patiently showed me programs thousands of times, until I finally
realized their significance.

CONTENTS

PART III

Some Implications and Applications

PREFACE

THE TITLE of this book may raise some eyebrows, even before the reader opens the cover. Can an author fairly propose to explain how the human brain works? Is not the brain unfathomable, baffling in its complexity, a mystery of mysteries?

The answer is a vigorous "no." The human brain will, to be sure, provide ample research problems for investigators for generations to come, but these will largely concern details and specific mechanisms. The main reason for this book is that the brain today is not merely comprehensible but, in general, very well understood by specialists in the field. Knowledge of its basic organization, role, functioning, development, evolution, and biological-electrical-chemical operation is both impressive and supported by a large accumulation of hard evidence.

As in most areas of technical study, knowledge has in recent decades not so much grown as exploded. The neuroscientists, finding or creating new tools, have used them for research with brilliant success. Discoveries and advances in contiguous fields have widened the foundation of understanding. Among the specialists, although they dispute vigorously on unresolved points, agreement on what can be called the "nature" of the human brain is broad and firm—certainly amply so for our present purposes.

But between the researchers and those who do not share their special worlds—and private languages—there exists a vast information gap, a veritable chasm. Worse, the whole subject of "brain" has long been clouded by outdated, mythical, popular concepts that could hardly be more wrong. Typically, the otherwise informed citizen, and even some more traditional academics and professionals in the "softer" disciplines, suffer from the classic problem: knowing too much that isn't so.

In our daily living and specific attempts to solve social problems, these misconceptions produce all too visibly an enormous amount of frustration, tension, failure, and conflict. We have been brought up with some grossly inaccurate ideas, and we tend to act on them. The results we get are what we might expect from applied nonsense—but where once we had serious mischief we now have threat to our very survival.

The time has come, I suggest, when we cannot afford not to understand the brain in modern terms, if we wish to understand ourselves or to deal effectively with people in our daily activities. This book is intended for all who have more than a casual interest in *what makes us behave as humans*, and especially for parents, educators, managers, communicators, planners, and all whose work involves human interactions.

I have come to this consideration of "brain" not as a scientist or a reporter on the neurosciences, but as an investigator of learning, that activity so peculiarly important in humans. I now marvel at my stupidity for years in not realizing what now seems so obvious: that learning is a brain function, and that trying to understand it is futile unless we first understand the brain.

Because I am not a specialist and have approached this study with practical, human concerns rather than narrow technical objectives, I have been free to draw from many fields, including evolution, anthropology, biology, ethology, computer science, brain-oriented modern psychology, and educational history and research. We are beginning to realize that if we are to understand man, *we must look at him as a whole*, within his social setting, rather than disassemble him in the laboratory. This book represents an effort at synthesis in that spirit and, I hope, proves more than just a summary of pertinent knowledge—useful as that might be.

In one sense, the title of this book is narrow. My concern is with the brain in health, in ordinary daily use, in our present society, and not with peripheral aspects, gimmickry, or science-fiction speculations. I see no reason why millions of people cannot know as much about the human brain as they know, say, about automobiles. Should this come to pass, our quality of life might improve sharply. Insight into how the brain works can open wide new doors to ameliorating some of our most pressing problems.

A work of synthesis must, by definition, be derivative. My debts, if detailed, would themselves fill a small volume; to attempt to give credit with any degree of fairness would entail endless digressions. The references and quotations will identify my principal sources, and those expert in various fields will readily identify others. Four very distinguished names in the neurosciences must be mentioned here, because I have been deeply influenced by their achievements: Pribram, Luria, Hebb, and MacLean. I hope I have not done their ideas violence in making use of them so freely.

The diagrammatic drawings of the brain that appear in the text are the work of my long-time associate Jacques Ducas.

I owe warm thanks also to the good friends who have encouraged this long effort and have listened to my ideas, read the manuscript in progress, and offered criticism and help in many ways.

LESLIE A. HART

New Rochelle, New York

PART I

The Incredible

Human Brain and

How We Got It

CHAPTER 1

The Rediscovery of the Brain

L ET US get on target right from the outset: we are human
because we have human brains. While our body facilitates our acting
as humans, it is the brain that makes us human.

We issue from the womb as a few helpless pounds of flesh, totally
unable to survive without constant attention. Some twenty years
later, if all goes reasonably well, we have become full-grown adults
able to cope with a complex world.

What we have learned in the meantime very largely determines the
kind of human each of us individually is—and that learning has
taken place *in the brain*, nowhere else.

What we sense—see, hear, feel, smell, taste—we sense *in the brain*,
nowhere else. As Dr. Ernest Gardner, dean of the Wayne State University School of Medicine, states in *Fundamentals of Neurology*,
"Perception is not possible until the impulses reach the brain."[1]
Only in the brain does the input have meaning; and then only as
we have individually learned to give it meaning; and even then only
as the brain chooses to receive and interpret what has been sensed
at all!

Our emotions arise *in the brain*, nowhere else—and they arise and
are controlled and expressed by the process (which we will examine

closely) we call "thinking." I put that word in quotation marks because its meaning is exceedingly vague. We use it to mean "whatever goes on in the brain."

If we acquire physical skills, they are *in the brain*, nowhere else.

Our plans, dreams, hopes, fears, goals, attitudes; ability to relate to other people, or circumstances or events; our love life, our life style, our bravery or timidity, confidence or anxiety—all this is almost purely a matter of brain, and almost all, by the time we are adult, has been learned. All the words we can speak, or read, or hear, and which give us the speech that is the most distinguishing mark of being human, have to be learned. We are by no means born as blobs or blank slates, but to an overwhelming degree *we are dependent on learning to become human, to think and feel and act as people*—which seems good enough reason for us to pay close attention to learning, including that sometimes sorry aspect of it called schooling or education.

Man is a brain freak. Among the more than one million species in the animal kingdom, his brain and its power of speech are unique. Even creatures without brains can learn, for learning and life itself were early linked. But man's brain reflects an enormous *need* to learn, because so much behavior is acquired, not innate; no other species begins to approach humans in individuality—which many people might agree is the essence of being human. We know a lot about what a rat or a dog or an ape will do, sight unseen, because there are fairly fixed rat, dog, or ape ways of behaving. But we cannot have the vaguest notion of how an unknown person will dress, or find food, or court, or even of how a mother will deal with her baby. These depend heavily on culture, which is to say on learning, which is to say—again—on the brain.

Yet in these days when man has, for the first time, the means of exterminating his species by pressing a few buttons, all too few people other than specialists have even a smattering of understanding of the nature of the human brain, in which such a decision would be made. And how much is known (in the sense of being useful) about the fostering of learning, the developing of confident individuals? Or of how, in brain terms, to get people to change so they can cope with change?

Lack of knowledge of the brain that actuates us probably does less damage than knowing too much that isn't so, most of it picked up as "psychology," surely the most befuddled of sciences. I must warn the reader who has been conventionally victimized in this way that much unlearning will be called for, if the modern information-processing approach is to be understood. Even such basic terms as "stimulus," "motivation," "conditioning," and "reinforcement" must be challenged as grossly misleading.

Many locutions and words in our common speech also contribute to fuzzing our ideas of how the brain functions. We may refer to the "trained fingers" of a concert pianist. The performer may have developed suitable muscles, but no training or learning has taken place in the hand—only in the brain. Should by misfortune the nerves that connect those fingers with the brain be severed, or a lesion in the brain prevent instructions from being sent or feedback from being received, the artist's skill will vanish instantly.

Emotions, too, are commonly spoken of as in the heart, or gut, or elsewhere. We are breathless with excitement, have no stomach for a quarrel, walk on air at good news. We talk of the "conflict between heart and head" as though emotion was somehow not brain activity but something separate and somehow opposite. Those who gave King Richard the title of Lion-Hearted were not merely being poetic —they would have been amazed that anyone doubted courage was seated in the heart. Around the turn of the century, William James and Karl Lange put forward an idea that became popular: that we felt "fear" because of and *after* physical responses such as shortening of the breath or running away—an ingenious but wrong interpretation. We can say with assurance today that emotions and emotional-control learning are wholly brain functions. Unless the brain evaluates a situation as calling for "emotional" response— essentially fight or flight, except for sex—the hormones that produce various bodily changes are not "ordered" into the bloodstream.

Some years ago, when experimenters found that electric probes precisely placed deep in cats' brains would produce all the responses of rage, they at first cautiously called it "sham rage." A number of such emotion centers have since been found and "sham" has been dropped. As we shall see, the relation of emotion to learning is of critical importance in understanding how the brain operates.

In a way, it is absurd that one should feel compelled to begin this discussion by flatly stating the dominance of the brain, but experience convinces me that not a few readers will boggle even at what has already been set down. The now-established view is hardly new. Twenty-five centuries ago Hippocrates, in *On the Sacred Disease,* taught that the brain had this all-controlling role. "From the brain and the brain alone arise our pleasures, joys . . . pains, griefs . . . through it we think, see, hear. . . ." One would think that endless experience with the wounds of war and accidents of peaceful living would constantly have reminded observers that the jellylike mass in the skull had essential control functions. Nor is it too easy not to observe that while our bodies in general have the bones inside and soft parts outside, the head reverses this and puts continuous armor all around the brain.

But as Greek thought went into eclipse with the fall of the Roman Empire, this understanding of the primacy of the brain gave way to weird and wonderful folklore. In part religious beliefs had influence: man had a soul, and "soul" and "mind" became confused. The soul departed at death, and therefore had to live somewhere in the body during life—the heart being one noble location. In the seventeenth century Descartes advanced the radical idea that the soul lived in and actuated the pineal "gland" in the brain. He was under the impression that only man, not animals, had such an organ. (Its function still uncertain, the pineal body may be a remake of what had once been a top eye or light receptor in man's evolutionary past and perhaps is now our internal "clock.")

At another period the brain was thought to be mainly a device for cooling the blood. Even more bizarre, perhaps, was the belief that it was merely a reservoir of mucus and that the common cold presumably caused some leakage. We can hope this hypothesis represented low ebb.

Today we might say that the brain is being rediscovered—faster in some quarters than in others. Public awareness that we have brains, that the brain is dominant, and that understanding it may be crucial is by all evidence—books, articles, television programs—growing rapidly. But in general, people have only the palest notion of the astounding achievements made by neuroscientists and by what we can term "primate and brain-oriented" psychologists (in contrast to the far greater number of "behaviorists").

Current neuroscience techniques are breathtaking in their delicacy, intricacy, and ingenuity, and ever more advanced investigative tools have accelerated progress at a dazzling rate. As will be apparent, I have drawn heavily on the resulting, massive body of well-established knowledge.

But outside the neuroscience area, great formless drifts of the old "nonbrain" psychology persist, and the term "psychology," especially in the United States, tends to refer to the now outworn but familiar part of the discipline. The enormously impressive and solidly based knowledge of the brain remains available rather than proffered. Much of it lies behind fences of formidable technical jargon that gives specialists themselves problems in communicating across disciplines. Those fragments that do enter major media may distort the picture, by being the more dramatic, bizarre, and sometimes alarming morsels that make better headlines—"brain control," biofeedback techniques, psychosurgery, chemical learning, and the like. What seems to be our great need—to acquire integrated, holistic, and fundamental concepts —tends to be poorly served. I have even encountered people who frankly say they are "afraid" of the brain—as though our happy, peaceful, and problem-free world would benefit by preserving ignorance.

One might expect, with the Hippocratic view of the brain's dominance fully restored and supported by hard evidence, that our educators would naturally be the most visible group at the head of an impatient line waiting for admission to the brain, as though it were a hit show. Astonishingly, we find just the opposite. From classroom teacher to college professor to the authors of those expensive, heavy books that education students must plow through on pain of banishment and noncertificatedness, lack of interest in the brain tends to be exceeded only by ignorance—spiced with misinformation—of what goes on within the skull.

If such a statement sounds incredible to the reader not closely acquainted with that vast enterprise, in many ways our largest, called "American education," let me merely refer him to the nearest library affording a reasonable sampling of educational literature—the latest included. Take from the shelves a few of those 400- or 500-page volumes titled "Educational Psychology" or the like, and consult their tables of contents and subject indexes. In many you will find no mention of the brain whatsoever,[2] in others reference to no more than a paragraph or a few pages. The paragraph is likely to remark that the brain is complex and not well understood. The few pages, which often give the impression that they have been stuck in as part of the "updating" of such texts, usually deal with some distinctly peripheral aspect of the brain.

Or turn to the current literature, in those dozens of trade publications and journals—some of high quality—that flood onto the educational scene, and again you will find, typically, that the word "brain" seldom appears, let alone any discussion that reflects recognition of its dominant importance.[3] Review the catalogs of colleges that presumably prepare millions for careers in education, training, personnel work, management, industrial engineering, journalism, and other occupations that require an understanding of what makes people human, and only rarely will you come on a course that studies the brain in any depth. Most likely the candidates will be obliged to wade through classical conditioning and Pavlov's dogs, Ebbinghaus's invention of the nonsense syllable, and innumerable accounts of starved rats.

Staggering as it seems, a wide chasm exists in education—using that term in its broadest sense—separating thought and behavior from the wellspring of their very being, the human brain. Subhuman animals do not have smaller human brains, but rather intellects that lack the characteristics that mean "human." Any psychology built on rats and pigeons more likely will mislead than help, especially if it ignores even these creatures' brains!

To dramatize the absurdity of our plight, try to imagine a large convention of automobile engineers, designers, production men, and managers, all deeply concerned with automobiles but all confessing that they know almost nothing about engines, drive trains, or engine controls. They explain that these areas are no doubt of great importance, but they are so complex that discussion will be avoided. "If you press down the gas pedal, the motor will turn over faster," an engineer explains. "We don't know why, but we don't want to go under the hood to find out."

Invite a handy tinkerer, perhaps one who has worked as an assembler in a television factory but who has no knowledge of electronics theory, to design and build a television receiver. Give him all the parts and tools he requests, and all facilities—and a hundred lifetimes. Without knowing what he is doing, without insight into "how it works," *without theory*, his chances of making a workable set by fit-and-try or luck are close to zero. In one way, the educators who play this game have even worse odds, for the "parts" they are working with and the "set" they are trying to build are constantly changing with the times, even as they try to fit pieces together.

Here and there some partial successes—and relative successes—do come to light, usually because of the intuitions and efforts of exceptional individuals. But without any viable theory as a foundation, these achievements have a nasty habit of crumbling away when no longer sustained by a charismatic or strong leader.

The need for a theory of learning that is *useful* in child rearing, formal education, training, and the whole range of "people" needs, and that is valid in its conception of the human brain, has become desperate. By general admission, nothing of the sort appears to be prominently available. Those instructing in schools, business, industry, the military, and elsewhere typically reject traditional "educational psychology" as of little or no use. New teachers taking on classroom duties overwhelmingly express this view.[4] (When schoolteachers do take an interest in some specific aspect of behaviorist psychology, it is usually to find some means of *controlling* students, of "making them behave," rather than to help them learn in the broader sense.)[5]

Many of the best-known educational psychologists are not too shy about confessing the lack of a useful, reasonably complete theory of learning applicable to human beings. In the introduction to one of the few general discussions of this topic, *The Psychology of Learning Applied to Teaching*, Dr. B. R. Bugelski states with impressive modesty:

> At the present time there is little to offer by way of practical advice to harassed teachers. Some psychologists would even argue that really there is nothing to say, and these will question the propriety of such a text as this. . . . Even if it were true that nothing of value can be stated about teaching, it would be worthwhile for teachers to learn that psychologists who have studied learning intensively do not really know much about the process.[6]

This view is endlessly repeated in the behaviorist literature on human learning—and it should be noted that many of the psychologists in the field see little or no distinction between a theory of "learning" and a theory of "behavior." (This is not a view I subscribe to quite so readily.) At times their language outdoes Professor Bugelski's for frankness. In an article on "The Scientific Study of Teacher Behavior," authors Donald M. Medley and Harold E. Mitzel remark:

> An honest appraisal of the content of teacher training would reveal that it does not resemble the rigorous quantitative set of laws which form the substance of the training of architects or engineers as much as it resembles the treasured store of traditions passed on by one witch doctor to another.[7]

The *Sixty-third Yearbook of the National Society for the Study of Education*, published in 1964, deals with *Theories of Learning and Instruction* and provides a broad review by many eminent contributors—with general agreement on the very modest usefulness of conventional theories of learning. In one chapter Professor Robert Glasser reviews the use of "principles of learning" derived from conventional psychology as applied in a quite different context: army training. Referring to the well known efforts of Robert M. Gagné, he notes Gagné's caution that the best-known principles prove "strikingly inadequate" for designing effective training situations.[8] While the military, going a very different route than schools and colleges, obtained some positive results by using such devices as flight simulators, these stemmed from an engineering systems or experiential approach far more than from any application of learning theory.

In *Toward a Theory of Instruction*, one of the very few books on this subject, Dr. Jerome Bruner of Harvard, whose ideas have done much to shake up the educational establishment, also notes that pedagogy depends principally on "a body of maxims." But he makes an additional point that too seldom is given attention:

> A theory of instruction, which must be at the heart of educational psychology, is principally concerned with *how to arrange environments to optimize learning* according to various criteria. . . (italics added).[9]

This observation has key importance. A theory of learning does not automatically produce a theory of instruction—or necessarily even a general theory of behavior. But certainly "maxims," "principles," or so-called theories that are fragmentary or do not apply to humans cannot serve as any adequate foundation for useful application theories.

The implications are horrendous: we pour out some $90 billion a year annually in the United States on schools and higher education;[10] we compel virtually every child to spend at least a dozen years —and often as many as twenty years—in the hands of educators; we set great store on diplomas and degrees; yet we see that in the deepest, most consequential sense educators in general do not know what they are doing, why they are doing it, or what they should be doing. We live in a technological society that needs an enormous amount of specialized training, yet we have blanks where we should have sound theory, and practice built on it, for producing the expertise we so sorely lack.

And we endure a jittery, crowded, frenetic yet often boring quality of life, with the lid barely holding down the violence that frequently spills through, without utilizing the available understanding of the human brain and behavior that might ease many of our most pressing problems—crime, alienation, poverty, disease, hate, and fear included.

CHAPTER 2

The Need to Make Sense

NO OUTCOME of our educational system is curiouser, to use Alice's term, than that "science" can be studied for ten to fifteen years without producing a grasp of the primacy of theory in today's world. Most of the food we eat, the clothes we wear, the shelter we occupy, the vehicles we move in, could not come into being by trial and error or by tinkering, but only by the application of theory—a deep, generalized understanding of the forces operating.

Yet the majority of officially educated Americans seem to show alarm at the mere mention of the word *theory*. Theory is viewed as something vague, impractical, remote, complicating.

The practical way to attack a problem, they will tell you, is to attack it directly. People don't behave the way you want them to? *Make* them behave! So we put people in prison to "teach them a lesson," and when they get out they promptly commit more crimes. We criticize or yell at or threaten those who displease us (if we can get away with it) but find they keep right on behaving the same way. Children don't learn or do what we wish, in or out of school, so we scold or punish them, with little effect (except bad effect), but we keep right on repeating the same futile efforts. Thousands of messages tell drivers to fasten their seat belts, but they don't. Somehow, the "practical," direct attack doesn't work too well. But we almost totally lack the alternative: valid and useful theory, the indirect way to gain grasp of the forces and principles that are at work.

The chapters that follow reflect an effort to collect, from a variety of fields of study, pertinent building blocks of available knowledge and to fit them unit by unit into a coherent, mutually supportive structure which has been given the name *Proster Theory.*

Some of this knowledge, a product of the last few years, has not had time to gain wide currency. Much more has been accessible for two or three dozen years, but only to those working within certain disciplines. (Specialists often lament the strictures of specializing and the difficulties of keeping abreast of developments in related fields; but they also exhibit "territoriality" more fiercely than robins, and tend to be shy about appearing to invade others' realms for fear of losing some plumage in instant attacks. Synthesizers must almost of necessity be nonspecialists, either foolish or daring enough to risk pleasing none of their sources.)

Building the Proster Theory in this discussion will involve excursions in a number of quite different directions—fortunately, mostly into fields of high inherent interest. Some patience must be asked of the reader as the blocks of knowledge are assembled and joined. It may be helpful to give some indication here of the theory that results.

It suggests that the whole vast riddle of brain, and of human nature and behavior, can be enormously simplified by the unifying device of the concept of programs, and programs grouped in bundles of alternatives termed *prosters.* (Proster is a neologism, obtained by compressing "program structure" to create a new word free of any old connotations.) The idea of programs is hardly new. For generations psychologists, even self-blindfolding behaviorists, have noted programs, often under such terms as "habits," "chains of behavior," "sequences," "goal-directed behavior," and more recently "plans." It is in fact difficult to observe animals in anything close to nonexperimental settings *without* soon seeing programs in some form. But often these observations were embarrassing to investigators, because they either did not fit in with, or indeed actively contradicted, theoretical approaches already under construction. Efforts to explain programs in stimulus-response terms resulted in absurdly complex structures. Practical wisdom and investigative convenience dictated that programs, like a hornet's nest, be noted but uninspected.

But on the brain side, we find two of the world's most eminent researchers explicitly identifying the concept of programs as a basic of brain function. The Soviet psychoneurologist A. R. Luria, professor of psychology at the University of Moscow, has stated flatly: "Modern psychological investigations have made it clear that each behavioral process is a complex functional system based on a plan or program of operation that leads to a definite goal."[1] Karl H. Pribram, research professor at the Stanford University School of Medicine, has been a pioneer in advancing understanding of the brain along similar lines, emphasizing programs, a hierarchic structure, "homeostats set in the context of other homeostats,"[2] and interconnected biasing—concepts I have adapted, with gratitude, in elaborating Proster Theory.

The advent of the computer brought both the term and concept *program* into common language use. As the computer industry catapulted forward, it sometimes happened that the expensive machines or "hardware" reached a customer well before the "software," or programs and related materials on paper, was ready. The equipment then sat, inert and useless, until the programs finally came—dramatically demonstrating their crucial importance.

The role of programs in brain functions tends to be concealed by complexities, the brain being a vastly more intricate and powerful apparatus than the largest computer. But Proster Theory holds that the human brain works by programs, and that when we begin to regard it from that viewpoint, its operations soon start to make sense even to the layman. The bits and pieces of knowledge from many sources suddenly fit together, and a basic organization appears. When we relate it to the brain's history, about which we know a good deal, what we can call the "nature" of the brain, as man's controlling, integrating organ, also emerges. It has a remarkably improbable structure, and utterly fantastic resources, but overall what it is and how it works becomes far more understandable.

To acquire this grasp of organization and function, we do not need to go deeply into such matters as the chemistry and physics of an impulse moving along a nerve, or the specific molecular changes involved in "engramming" memories. Brain scientists in a long list of disciplines will be busy with solving technical problems for perhaps a century to come, at least. In the meantime, we can take advantage of what is known, consolidated into a theory, to better understand relations among people, and to increase insight into ourselves.

We can acquire some confidence in the theory by checking it two contrasting ways: by verifying that it remains consistent with the current knowledge of the brain's physiology, and by comparing what the theory tells us about humans with what we observe about common human behavior.[3] If Proster Theory fits reasonably well both ways, it can have immediate usefulness, even though, as is usual with broad theories, time may bring many refinements and corrections.

Theories of this nature—perhaps they can be called the "order out of chaos" type—are often quite simple. For example, Dalton gave chemistry a huge advance by his concept of atoms as indestructible bits of matter that combined in an orderly way, an idea improved by Avogadro, and then carried into Mendeleev's periodic table of elements and the modern image of the atom as a nucleus with rings of electrons. These ideas, heavily speculative as they were at first, suggested to those working in the field where to look and what to look for. They were organizing ideas that brought the bits and pieces together; and because the bits and pieces often fitted nicely, and matched observed reality, the theory had great practical usefulness. Mendeleev's table, in fact, permitted predicting the nature of many elements not then known.

In much the same way Darwin and Wallace, independently observing that species appeared to adapt by gradual small changes, brought order out of the confusion that then existed, even though many aspects of evolutionary mechanisms still occasion debate and further research. Mendel's work on heredity offers another classic example: his findings on traits were in essence very simple, yet so powerful an organizing concept that the doors to the science of genetics swung wide open. Nor can we forget Copernicus and Galileo, whose basic idea was that the earth goes around the sun, not the sun around the earth as our senses plainly tell us. Although their supportive observations were complex, the organizing concept was simple enough to put in one sentence.

Proster Theory, in this general pattern, is an effort to find a relatively simple organizing concept that will fit the best facts we have. If it does, even moderately well, it can immediately have usefulness in some of the "people" areas that most concern us today, from rearing children or hiring employees to preventing war or relieving individual mental problems. "Brain," as more writers are beginning to point out, is one of our last great frontiers.[4] Well-educated people commonly have less correct knowledge of it than the contemporaries of Copernicus had of the solar system.

Because a program approach to the brain has been so inadequately explored in the past, except by specialists, it may take us on some unfamiliar paths. It calls for discarding many ideas as "obviously true" as that the world is flat and the sun goes around it. For instance, we have to deal with a brain that is enormously, aggressively active, not the responder to stimuli that conventional psychology has induced many to believe. We will have to deal with such (probably) startling findings as this, by Luria, in *The Working Brain*:

> To the unprejudiced observer, *musical hearing and speech hearing* may appear to be two versions of the same psychological process. However, observations on patients with local brain lesions show that destruction of certain parts of the left temporal region leads to a marked disturbance of speech hearing (discrimination between similar sounds of speech is completely impossible), while leaving musical hearing unimpaired. . . . This means that such apparently similar mental processes as musical hearing and speech hearing not only incorporate different factors, but also depend on the working of quite different areas of the brain.[5]

The difficulties inherent in shifting to a radically new organizing viewpoint may perhaps be seen more sharply if we imagine ourselves the shifter rather than the one who must shift.

Suppose you penetrate the jungles of central Brazil and find a member of an isolated tribe that has never heard of radio. You place your portable before him, snap the power switch, select short-wave, turn up the volume, tune to a station. Music issues from the speaker. To your tribesman this appears incredible to the point of magic. You move the dial and speech comes forth. More magic!

Your tribesman is intelligent and sensible. He suspects *you* of producing the effect. You move a hundred yards away. Now he reasons that there must be tiny people in the box. You return, remove the back, show him the circuitry inside. For him, the mystery deepens.

As familiarity replaces initial fear, your tribesman may learn to operate the controls, finding different stations and turning the volume up or down. He has utterly no notion, of course, of what he is doing, or why he sometimes gets music or talk and other times nothing. The behavior of the box at first appears totally unpredictable; later a few patterns emerge—he can see, for example, that the dial has to be at a certain spot, the SW switch on, and the volume turned up to get music. But at other times, the same procedure produces talk, and at still other times, when the station is off the air, nothing but a buzz.

Other tribesmen might well try looking inside the box, too. You might hear your friend tell them there is no use in doing so, since the inside is incomprehensible—precisely what most behaviorist (and some other) psychologists have long told one another with respect to the brain.

No matter how long the tribesman plays with the controls or how carefully he observes what happens as he experiments, he can never come to understand what is actually happening, nor really grasp what the controls do. In fact, if you were now to tell him that there are broadcasting stations in many distant cities, that they send out imperceptible waves that carry the signal, and that the tuner, in either AM or SW mode, enables the box to match and pick up the waves, which are then transduced to sound, he will reject this outrageous nonsense.

New theories, especially if valid, usually sound absurd at first blush: tiny invisible creatures cause many diseases; fossils are remains of life forms that existed millions of years ago; a few pounds of a certain chemical, brought into one mass, can blow a large city off the face of the earth. The history of science consists of a long series of such outrageous nonsensical pronouncements—including a multitude that turned out to *be* nonsense.

Let us assume that you are able to take your friend the tribesman to a laboratory, where over a period of time you manage to convince him that signals can be sent over a wire, and then without the wire. Next you introduce him to radio stations and their activities. With patience, you may bring him to see your explanation as acceptable.

Now he can make sense of the magic box. He knows that snapping the switch to "on" sends power from the batteries to the transistors, and so forth. He may still have knowledge gaps, such as why the transistors function as they do, but he now has broad insight into what is happening, and to a degree that insight replaces magic, folklore, tradition, and mystification. His ability to control the radio, to make it function well, has gained enormously. If the switch does not turn on the power, he can suspect a cell is out of place and adjust it so the batteries are again supplying energy. If a station comes in weakly, he can rearrange the antenna—still with a certain amount of trial and error, but guided by understanding of what is operating. If a station is "off the air," he knows why he cannot receive it.

In our general efforts to produce learning, to educate, to train people for work, and to influence behavior of people at all ages, we resemble the tribesman tinkering with the knobs—except that in our task far more knobs present themselves, with many changing shape and function even as we try to manipulate them. We may be almost unaware of the far distant "stations" that still send signals from our evolutionary past, and we understand little about what is on the other, hidden end of the controls, and the rest of the "works" in this box of bone. A suitable theory of learning, of how the brain functions, serves above all else to help us understand what we are doing and what is operating.

Surrounded by machines whose innards are unknown territory, like blank spaces on a map, most of us at one time or another have succumbed to frustration and given the offending, recalcitrant device a swift kick. Once in a while the tactic works: the television produces a picture, or the soft drink machine disgorges a bottle. More usually we only stub our toe and leave a dent. It seems worthwhile to point out that children and adults are frequently kicked in similar frustration.

The path to humane education and interpersonal relations follows understanding. It is not enough to mean well. The surgeon who excises an appendix rates as no less kindly or sympathetic because he knows what he is doing.

Most "educational" effort, I submit, ranges from a mild to a severe, crippling form of continuous torture for the students. As we shall discuss, the institutions established and the methods widely used in them fight human nature at every turn. Teachers and administrators, trainers and bosses, officials and legislators usually do not mean to be cruel, but the evidence shows overwhelmingly that in effect they are. As a consequence, we live in an age of long-overdue rebellion.

Proster Theory, however mechanistic our approach to it may seem, may conceivably help to create institutions and ways of treating people that are consistent with their nature and their needs, their growth as healthy and confident personalities, and their productive use of the astonishing brains they were endowed with.

CHAPTER 3

Psychology: A Rat-Burdened Science

HOW DID so appalling a chasm develop between our need to understand human learning and behavior on the one hand, and the disciplines of psychology and education on the other? Why is psychology, which as an experimental science is at least a hundred years old, of such little use to us in daily life? How is it possible that education, with such massive financing, popular support, and armies of workers, usually operates like something out of the fifteenth century—crude, primitive, wasteful, ineffective, destructive in its resistance to needed change?

How conceivably did many psychologists (the exceptions are most important, of course) get so far off the track of reality and into ever more complex futilities, like spiders weaving webs in a sealed glass case? And what is the explanation for educators pretending the human brain does not exist, insofar as they show such little recognition of its nature?

To answer these questions would take at least one book in itself; here I can offer no more than a few hints. At the beginning of this century, psychology was a fairly young and wobbly field of study desperately trying to become a respectable science—behaving much like a social climber from a declassé background. Psychology indeed had a lot to get disentangled from. The work of Franz Gall and Johann Spurzheim, while on a fruitful track, had led to the elaborate and widely publicized nonsense of phrenology—the notion that the shape of the skull reflected bents and capacities; the locution "a large bump of curiosity," for example, remains in common language. Enormous interest in the "animal magnetism" of Franz Mesmer, the eighteenth-century physician and hypnotist who in turn had been inspired by astrological beliefs of Paracelsus, favored the blossoming interest in hypnosis. In investigating this phenomenon, the great early neurologist Jean Charcot attracted Sigmund Freud, whose work deriving from the use of hypnosis soon began to shake and horrify the polite world, not at all accustomed to having s-e-x said aloud, let alone considered important in childhood.

Over these public excitements lay the thick mixture of elusive concepts long associated with "mind." Religion, soul, mysticism, folklore, philosophy, and quackery were all ingredients of this stew. Even today, "mind" remains the beautifully vague word used by many, if not most, psychologists and educators at all levels to camouflage the largest gaps in their systems. Centuries ago personality was supposed by learned men to reflect the individual mixture of "humors" or fluids: blood (sanguine), yellow bile (choleric, bilious), black bile (melancholic) and phlegm (phlegmatic); we still speak of "being in a good humor." "Mind" is a term perhaps a little *less* scientific than these. We find it used as copiously as "brain" is not, and such use should at once alert our suspicions.

Much as many people rebelled against Darwin's efforts to look at the origin of humans and other species realistically—and were appalled that divine man could be merely another animal—so we still have those who feel more comfortable with "mind," and cringe at the invitation to look at man's brain in evolutionary terms. At the beginning of the century, of course, religious pressures were far greater than today. "Mind" graciously sheltered "soul," while "brain" might prove to be a harsh landlord who would turn soul out into the cold. For those who took soul seriously and literally, any investigation of brain was threatening.

We may doubt that many investigators today hesitate to disturb the kind of soul that could flutter to Heaven on pigeon wings; in any case, where literal Heaven used to be we now have Space, with satellites, laboratories, and military spy-eyes whizzing around. "Mind" finds such frequent use because it is much handier to say or write one four-letter word than the awkward six words of "that which I do not understand." If we grasp the meaning, we can surely forgive the shortcutting. Thousands of hours could be saved annually in lectures alone.

What psychology needed at the turn of the century was something that looked, sounded, and if possible smelled "scientific," as if it had escaped from a physics or chemistry lab. The great Ivan Petrovich Pavlov appeared on cue, with the prestige of a Nobel Prize (awarded in 1904 for studies, as a physiologist, of digestive juices). Pavlov performed his famous conditioned reflex experiments on dogs, producing delightfully hard evidence that scientists in more respectable fields could hardly dismiss with a sneer. "I measure," declared Pavlov. (Ironically, in later years he was criticized for theorizing about the brain as an entity, along lines that would be considered modern and on target today.)

Pavlov's work overlapped that of John B. Watson, who probably had the greatest role in setting American psychology on fruitless paths. Picking up broadly from John Locke, David Hartley (one of the first "associationists," born in 1705), and to a degree the eminent William James, Watson took an extreme position on the age-old nature/nurture controversy, favoring the viewpoint that a child is born as a "blank slate." This *tabula rasa* concept was a splendidly simple way out of the old "mind" confusion. If a newborn child was so much clay, to be shaped by conditioning, psychologists—and educators—could assume full control.

Watson studied infants for a time, seeking to prove his theory. But work on the conditioned reflex discovery (its importance enormously exaggerated) did not call for humans, who make awkward, expensive, slow-growing, and complicated subjects. Animals obviously made laboratory experimenting much easier, cheaper, and faster.

Usually, the first step was to put the animal in some form of captivity, in the best "scientific" tradition of simplifying and controlling the conditions and variables. This of course ignored the plain fact that all higher animals have brains developed to deal with complex conditions in a state of freedom, not with strange, unnatural boxes in a state of confinement. But we must remember that the psychologist, intent on gaining a doctoral degree or publishing a paper, perhaps, very seldom had the slightest interest in the animal as an animal, as a living whole. It was simply a small sample of mind to be subjected to various bizarre tests, as one might take samples of chemicals and make tests with heat or acid or catalysts to see what happened, and with good luck, to get a yes-or-no answer to an hypothesis. The ethological approach, to observe what animals themselves did in a natural environment, has come to the fore only recently, at least in the United States. (Even ethologists, anthropologist David Pilbeam has pointed out, may at times be too hasty in accepting conditions as "natural".)[1] In brief, the general practice came to be to tear the subject animal apart, either surgically or psychologically, or both ways.

The favorite animal for the purpose became the laboratory rat, a white, pink-eyed rodent soon thousands of generations removed from existence in any natural world. Reared under conditions that we today know virtually guarantee extreme stupidity, it is about as close as we can get to a living nonanimal. Further, to "motivate" these albino victims, experimenters customarily severely starve them before dropping them into their mazes or puzzle boxes, with the result that experiments then deal with weakened, probably terrified creatures fighting for survival. From the behavior of test animals under such conditions, conclusions are drawn about "mind," which often end up, in spite of weak warnings, being applied to human behavior. (The noted Dr. B. F. Skinner likes to use pigeons, creatures far off man's evolutionary path. He then writes books seemingly suggesting humans can be managed as if they were pigeons.)

Work with humans has long comprised a small proportion of the total effort. And even when people were used as subjects, they tended to be either very young or college students—these being the easiest to work with or most conveniently available. Indeed, *convenience* has had an enormous influence on what psychologists have chosen to do. This tendency is frequently acknowledged by psychologists themselves. For example, in *Learning, Language and Cognition*, Arthur W. Staats observes quite typically:

> The field of experimental psychology of learning has largely been a morass of theoretical controversy and unorganized experimentation —from the standpoint of the person who is interested in understanding significant human behaviors.[2]

In *Introduction to Modern Behaviorism* Howard Rachlin laments that psychologists

> favor piecemeal attacks on specific areas of behavior, for which they use whatever tools are convenient and effective.[3]

I do not mean to imply that psychologists are unique in this respect. Einstein expressed distaste for scientists who choose to drill investigative holes in a piece of wood where the wood is thinnest, and René Dubos, in *So Human an Animal*, notes that scientists "shy away from the problems posed by human life" because they are not amenable to orthodox and familiar techniques of study, and refers to their "strange assumption that knowledge of complex systems will inevitably emerge from studies of much simpler ones."[4] Nor do I mean to ignore the many brilliant contributions that individual psychologists have made along the way or the investigators who have refused to cling to early Pavlovian approaches, now broadly conceded to be sterile and of little use in understanding more complex aspects of learning and behavior.

But overall, American academic psychology has been dominated by stimulus-response (S-R) and behaviorist investigations, working with subhuman and subprimate creatures, with fractions rather than entities, in T-mazes and Skinner boxes instead of realistic settings, and outside the skull rather than inside.[5] Significantly, the work of Jean Piaget, who closely observed real children in real surroundings (and whose name is now fashionably on the lips of any educator who is at all "with it"), attracted attention in the United States only after decades of delay. The ethologists only more recently have come to the fore. By and large, a hundred years of psychology has contributed little of organized or unified usefulness in understanding humans. Even the standardized testing that for a time seemed to hold great promise has come under deep suspicion, as often more misleading and damaging than helpful.

One tremendous factor, of course, and one that would be most unfair to ignore, was the lack of knowledge of the brain that prevailed during much of the present century. Those who tried to get inside the skull more often than not found themselves on very tenuous ground, and so a tradition of staying outside developed. But in the past three decades or so, progress in the brain sciences has been spectacular. Greatly improved electron microscopy techniques permit sharp pictures with magnifications of 50,000 diameters and more. (Even 500,000 is possible, but seldom wanted.) Brain structure can be *seen*—even the junctions between neurons, the synapses that the pioneering neurophysiologist Sir Charles Scott Sherrington, born in 1859, theorized must be there (they look much like adjoining button mushrooms). Huge advances in molecular biology and neural chemistry have opened up new understandings and pathways for further investigation of nerve and synapse functions. Incredibly small microelectrodes can now be placed accurately into single neurons, and the effect of receptor stimulation traced along nerve pathways—with some surprising results. Computers, coupled to sensitive brain-wave devices, can ferret out data previously hidden. The neurological apparatus of emotions has been clarified, producing some astounding demonstrations, such as cats terrified at the sight of mice. Medically necessary operations on humans, including even splitting the brain into two separate sides, have added to the knowledge long gathered from observation of wounds and other traumas. In the fields of genetics, evolutionary history (long almost totally ignored by psychologists), ethology, and anthropology, rich gains have been made in defining the role of the brain, its nature, and its functioning. The list could be easily expanded.

But (to generalize again) psychologists have been slow, and educators far slower, to respond to these findings and to others derived from increased experimentation with primates such as chimpanzees, and from observation of "whole," not fractionated, animal and human behaviors. We can hazard a guess as to the two main reasons: first, the findings require abandoning many nonsensical ideas that were long taken seriously; and second, psychologists, even some of the more advanced, find it extremely difficult to abandon outworn words and methods (programs) they were brought up with—or even to see how severely they are handicapped by terms such as "stimulus" or "reinforcement" that at once distort and confuse. One of the most widely known American psychologists, Professor J. McVicker Hunt, has added a touch of irony by pointing out that "It is precisely observations from S-R methodology which have undone traditional peripheral S-R theory, and it is these observations which are now demanding that brain function be conceived in terms of active processes."[6]

As for the cobwebbed world of education, one can only share the outrage of the distinguished Dr. Herbert A. Thelen, who a few years ago said bluntly:

> I think our present situation is grave; more, it is immoral. For to act ignorantly when knowledge is available, to deny realities that patently exist and make a general difference is the worst crime of civilized man.[7]

American behaviorist and S-R psychology has led us terrifyingly far off solid ground into a "morass,"[8] while education has not led us at all. For a century clearer-sighted, less herd-bound individuals have struggled to get back on a productive track. A function of this book is to bring together much of their thinking and findings, and the newer discoveries, so as to suggest at least an approach and direction. But to move ahead, we must shake off antiquated ideas and methods as we turn to humans and the human brain.

CHAPTER 4

A Brain to Learn With

THE HUMAN BRAIN is the organ of the body that occupies the upper part of the head, fitting into a sturdy container of bone. The brain can be measured, weighed, probed, dissected, examined microscopically, and subjected while alive to various examinations, treatments, sectioning, and excisions. It is as specific as "mind" is vague.

How old is man's brain? That depends of course on how we define "man." We have to turn to paleoanthropology for estimates that, if not overly precise, at least give us an idea to go by, subject always to some exciting new finding of fossil and cultural remains which can push dates further back. With present dating methods based on chemical or radioactive analysis, in addition to many earlier techniques, the dating of specific remains is far from guesswork.

Modern man—a term we can use to mean people substantially like those who dominate the earth today—has clearly existed at least 40,000 years. Recent discoveries may bring acceptance of an estimate of 120,000 years. Cro-Magnon man, best known to us as the painter of superb pictures in French caves, loosely means modern man during the hunting and gathering, pre-agricultural stage. Our first impression, were we to encounter one today, would be of a remarkably handsome, sturdy, and impressive person. The stereotype of cave man usually refers to Neanderthal man, who lived at least 100,000 years ago.

Neanderthals got their brutish reputation because the first major find, in a German quarry near Düsseldorf, came a bit too early. The year was 1856, three years before Darwin published *On the Origin of Species*, and the discovery of human remains obviously tens of thousands of years old was exceedingly awkward and upsetting to a society that preferred to take the biblical Genesis literally. Emotionally, it was easy for many who tried to face the hard facts of the find to brutalize the creature, to see the race as close to the ape, and so push Neanderthal away from present civilized man—much as one might wish to minimize the close relationship of a loutish cousin who suddenly turned up in town. The falsified description has lingered on, supported by reiterated errors, persisting embarrassingly long even in scientific literature. Neanderthal man did tend to have a receding chin and sloping forehead, and a little more hair on the chest and limbs than most males today, but he also had a larger cranium than a good share of the present population (not that brain size in itself means that much). Many specialists believe that a typical male specimen, shaved and dressed, could walk down Fifth Avenue today without exciting any particular attention.

Other races of early *Homo sapiens*, the species to which we belong and the only one to survive to the present, take the record back another 100,000 years. It seems safe to say, on the basis of remains already found, that *Homo sapiens* existed a quarter of a million years ago.

But the first man of our own genus, *Homo erectus*, who used tools and fire and maintained communities, takes us back three times as far. Beyond this rough 750,000-year point, the record indicates beings more appropriately called "manlike," although they stood and walked erect, used their hands much as we do and certainly used at least primitive tools. *Australopithecus*, considered by present knowledge the first definite hominid, was in all probability in existence two million years ago; and since there is a long gap in the record, a guess of four or five million would be reasonable.[1] *Ramapithecus*, a creature we would probably have had to look at twice to distinguish from what we think of as ape in terms of face, hair, and long arms, is usually called man's oldest ancestor of which we have some positive detail. This manlike primate takes us back some twelve to fifteen million years.[2]

We can conservatively assume, then, that the *Homo sapiens* brain has been in use some 250,000 years, and that brains with strongly human characteristics have been guiding behavior for a couple of million years—with development going forward in erect-walking primates for at least ten million years prior to that. Although such a period hardly amounts to much in the broad evolutionary context, it does imply that our brain is not quite a new apparatus, and it puts recorded history—a good deal less than 10,000 years—in perspective, as a time so brief as scarcely to matter.

But of course even the *Ramapithecus* brain, recent in the evolutionary sense, had behind it at very minimum half a billion years of unbroken development, extending back to the earliest appearance of nerve tissue in the earliest forms of life in our line of origin.[3]

To understand clearly how our evolutionary history affects the nature of our brain, and so our behavior every second of life, we must focus on the concept of need. Evolution can be thought of as a shaking-out or winnowing-down process that stresses the differences among individuals composing a species. To dramatize an extremely slow process, visualize a town of some 10,000 people suddenly uprooted by war or natural calamity. Initially their survival demands the ability to run rapidly for half a mile. Next, the people must swim a broad river and scale a steep cliff. Far fewer than the original number reach the top after these trials. A long trek over high mountain trails follows, eliminating many, especially those who have poor tolerance for cold. Coming to a warmer jungle, survivors now require a resistance to the stings of certain insects and exposure to certain diseases. Not many get through. But we can see that it was the variety of attributes that increased the odds that some would endure. Had none been able to swim, had all been susceptible to the jungle illnesses, the entire population would have been wiped out—and left no progeny.

If those who remain breed, their numbers soon increase, assuming favorable conditions. But the trials they went through will have narrowed down the kinds of genes they most often pass on.

If we think of this selection process continuing over very long periods, we can see "need" as having two quite different meanings, both critically important. On one hand, the attributes must fit the conditions existing at any one time sufficiently well to permit survival and reproduction on a scale that will perpetuate the species. On the other, the species must have, in some form, latent adaptability to meet *changing* conditions.

The prime mechanism of adaptability is not individual but species-wide, in the variability of individuals. For example, if individuals within a certain species of insects are almost identical, a change in the environment that negatively affects any may affect all and wipe them out. But if some vary from the norm considerably in size, shape, color, energy, or behavior patterns, it is far more likely that a minority will survive. Which will be able to survive the change to new conditions depends on each circumstance—the largest and strongest under the old conditions may be the first to be squeezed out if the new environment sharply reduces food supply, favoring those who don't require as much. In a region that becomes industrialized and smoggy, moths slightly darker than most may become less vulnerable to enemies because they are harder to see at rest.[4] In our present world, our aroused awareness of ecological problems makes it easy to see that clever, industrialized populations may poison themselves out of existence, while "backward" ones, in their ignorance of radioactivity and industrial wastes, hang on for the very reason that they are not as advanced.

Nature became more sophisticated, so to speak, with experience, moving from the kind of species adaptability, which does not involve learning, to individual adaptability that does. Even very simple forms of life (relatively speaking—even one-cell creatures can prove bewilderingly complex organisms) show some learning capacity. But reptiles and insects, in contrast to humans, behave in exceedingly rigid, repetitive patterns. They cling to what has worked for countless generations before them. Clearly such patterns have long met the needs of survival. They are passed on to the next generation not by any kind of teaching, but by genetic structure—they are built in. The ant behaves in a certain way for precisely the same reason that it has a certain typical shape of head, or kind of eye, or system of digestion.

This point has great importance to our present argument, in more than one way.

We cannot study or even observe the creatures around us without finding ample evidence that behaviors are passed on this way—genetically. A fish does not have to be taught an elaborate courting sequence. A bird "knows" how to build a nest. A dog circles before he lies down and wags his tail to convey pleasure and friendliness with no instruction or example whatever. Years ago ants and bees were presented as admirable examples of industry and good citizenship (many of us can remember this from our own school days), but today we recognize that they simply execute, on cue, programs that are as wired-in as the circuits of an amplifier.

In *The Machinery of the Brain*, Dean E. Wooldridge gives many examples of built-in, inflexible, stored programs of behaviors and offers the caution:

> Although observations such as those just described show conclusively that learning from experience is not occurring, the inheritance at birth of such detailed and purposeful behavior patterns is so different from anything we humans experience that it is necessary for us to fight against the tendency to imagine that reasoning intelligence is involved.[5]

As we come to the more recent, more elaborate forms of life, we find that while built-in behaviors continue to be transmitted, the more sophisticated capacity of learning after birth becomes increasingly apparent.

The amount of learning that is possible can vary along a continuum from almost none to the virtually unlimited extreme represented by modern man. But if the newborn creature is to learn, it must be "unfinished" at birth to a corresponding degree—for learning takes time and requires that the areas in the brain where the learning is to be stored be uncommitted or "plastic." For analogy, clay can be molded until it is baked. Once fired, it is committed to that shape. To quote Lionel Tiger and Robin Fox in *The Imperial Animal*:

> As we go up the phylogenic scale of mammals, we find several trends: life span increases; the gestation period becomes longer; the period of immaturity lengthens; the suckling period is extended; the size of the litter decreases until single births are most common. All these factors conspire to delay the maturity of the young animal as long as possible, to prevent his becoming fully formed too quickly.[6]

There is no sharp dividing line, of course, between "can't learn" and "can learn." As I have already noted, we find some evidence of ability to learn far down the evolutionary scale, even among creatures that have no nervous systems at all. We are dealing with a continuum and to some degree a trade-off. As learning capacity increases, there tends to be a decreasing reliance on built-in programs. To assume, however, that because modern man has relatively huge learning power, nothing remains of species learning or built-in behavior would be to make a very large jump indeed.

We should note, too, that the built-in factors do not have to be all-or-none. For example, a songbird can typically sing its characteristic, built-in song even if it has never heard another bird. But it will not sing as well, nor have the variations and repertoire of a similar bird that has been allowed to hear older birds sing. As we go up the phylogenic scale to more advanced, brainier creatures, we also find that the built-in programs, which can be exceedingly precise in insects or reptiles, tend to become patterns, allowing increasing room for variation. As patterns become still more diffuse, we can call them simply tendencies—but they may greatly influence our behavior.

In evolutionary terms, what is the "purpose" of permitting learning after birth to displace species wisdom? Plainly, the ability to learn more not only adds to species adaptability, but also allows the individual more room to adapt, and quickly. The darker moths survived, but the lighter ones got picked off by enemies. An individual moth had no power to adapt. But learning ability not only allowed man as species to adapt to changing conditions, but also gave the individual considerable latitude within a single lifetime.

This learning was for survival. The earth we inhabit constantly changes as an environment. Continents shift, collide, and thrust up mountains. Climates change. Sea level has risen and fallen. Roughly about the time that modern man's direct ancestors lived, the world's climate began to oscillate quite violently, producing a series of ice ages.[7] Swings from hotter to colder and back again enormously affected climate, sea level, and physical features. Even though such cycles could take tens of thousands of years, they often must have forced early man to move—and perhaps also invited him to by opening up new land bridges or routes through previous obstacles. Those who did not move as climate changed probably perished.

It seems most reasonable to suppose that among both the primates who were our precursors and early man there were variations in learning ability and in willingness to move, with the two attributes likely overlapping a good deal. Most creatures simply die out when changes in their habitat exceed what they can adapt to. The concept that "somewhere there may be a better living" is so abstract that only the top grade of brain can entertain it; and at first pre-men probably moved only under the pressures of imminent starvation. To survive even briefly in a new habitat called for exceptional learning ability; presumably those who had it to a higher degree survived more often, while those who lacked it succumbed. Subsequent generations inherited the ability.

Evolution normally proceeds as an extremely slow process, from our human point of view. Mutations, or genetic changes that seem to be induced by external energy sources, seldom occur, and the vast majority "don't work" and so are phased out. For a successful mutation to spread into many individuals' genes takes a great number of generations. Millions of years ordinarily were required to produce major change in most creatures.

The development of man's brain seems a startling exception. *Australopithecus'* brain averaged about 500 cubic centimeters, an impressive size achieved over tens of millions of years. But very soon thereafter (perhaps three to five million years) *Homo erectus* had cranial capacity about twice as great, with extremes at least up to 1,300 cubic centimeters—more than some present-day individuals may have.[8] Some evolutionists use the term "explosion" to express their awe at the rapidity of this change. *Something* caused it. Probably a number of factors combined to make ability to learn a strongly selective survival attribute; and likely these included the widespread effects of ice ages, some of which began or ended quite abruptly— in hundreds rather than thousands of years. The last terminated quite sharply a mere 12,000 years ago. The next, many scientists suspect, may be no more than 2,000 years in the future, and possibly pollution could hurry it along.

Two other related factors almost certainly played their part: man's equally explosive development of tool use, and his progress as a hunter of larger and more dangerous game.

Absorbing as exploration of man's past may be, we must confine our interest here to those aspects that throw some light on learning. The fossil and archeological record appears to make the key point abundantly clear: ability to learn had tremendous survival value for the evolutionary line that led to *Homo sapiens*—us.

Almost equally important is a second point: In spite of our "sudden" new need to be individual learners, we did not suddenly get new brains. We enlarged the old ones. There was no break with the past—no such break is possible in evolution. Our human brain has been in gradual development for half a billion years. We can hope to understand it only in that light.

CHAPTER 5

Man, the Brain Freak

WORDS have their own intrinsic potency. In the field of learning psychology, great mischief is made by some of the most common terminology, the worst culprits being, by my nomination, "stimulus," "conditioning," "reinforcement," "reward and punishment," and not least, "motivation."

These serve as the very keystones of the various American systems that collectively (not coherently) dominate most of the investigation that goes on in relation to learning. Since they all have acquired connotations that like twisted signposts point unfailingly the wrong way, their crippling effect is even greater than their use. The terms still confuse and misdirect even though evidence abounds that they should be largely abandoned.

Consider "motivation." References to motivation sprinkle educational and training literature, particularly that pertaining to the practice of teaching; and almost always the implication is negative. "Arthur could do much better," the teacher tells the parent, "but he doesn't seem to be motivated." The term sounds so respectable and familiar that a moment of thought may be needed to see that it fails to mean anything. Indeed, in J. P. Chaplin's *Dictionary of Psychology*,[1] a useful and often brutally frank handbook, motivation is defined as an "intervening variable which is used to account for factors within the organism which arouse, maintain, and channel behavior toward a goal." In further discussion, Chaplin notes that the concept is "among the most controversial and least satisfactory;" and astutely lists no less than twenty-six related terms, from "appetite" to "wish," that the reader might care to consult—presumably if sufficiently motivated toward trying to figure out what the term does or does not mean.

As far as learning is concerned, tremendous resistance seems to arise within many psychologists and educators at all levels to the simple notion that a child is *born* motivated to learn, and that he or she does not have to be pushed or manipulated in some fashion to comply with inner, personal, natural needs.

Picture my neighbor and me standing in a tulip bed in February. "I have planted fifty tulips here," I inform him. "How can I motivate them to come up in spring?"

The question is, of course, absurd in such a context. My tulips need proper planting, reasonably good soil, and the heat that warmer weather will bring. I can "*de*motivate" them in a number of ways— by piling a foot of earth on the bed, or putting down a planked flooring, or spreading various chemical agents. But the motivation to grow is *in* the bulbs. So are the precise instructions as to how to form leaves and construct the blossoms. These will have yellow flowers and these red, this variety will appear early and those nearly a month later. Whether they will be "motivated" to have tall stems or short, smooth petals or ragged, shallow cups or deep, has already been decided.

In *The Slow Learner in the Classroom* Newell C. Kephart makes the point succinctly:

> We cannot think of learning as something which is turned on or turned off at specific times, *as in a school classroom.* Learning is a dynamic factor in every activity of the organism (italics added).[2]

Dr. Kephart identifies the main issue in motivation as the word is most often used in education—applied not to learning as a continuing process of life, but to doing what the teacher directs, when and as directed, and stopping when told to. If I instruct my tulips to bloom on a certain Sunday because company is coming, I could expect results about as reliable.

Dr. Donald O. Hebb, one of the most eminent and productive pioneers among brain-oriented psychologists, and chancellor of McGill University, long ago expressed vigorous views on this point:

> The energy of response is not in the stimulus. It comes from the food, water, and oxygen ingested by the animal. . . . Any organized process in the brain is a motivated process, inevitably, inescapably; . . . the human brain is built to be active, and . . . as long as it is supplied with adequate nutrition will continue to be active. Brain activity is what determines behavior, and so the only behavioral problem becomes that of accounting for *in*activity.[3]

Learning, in humans, can readily be blocked, impeded, discouraged, or fostered, facilitated, encouraged—as we hardly need a specialist to tell us. But the one thing we don't have to do is motivate.

If we weren't motivated by a billion years of evolution to be learners, a few of us would be fossils of an extinct species and the rest of us would never have been conceived.

"*Cogito, ergo sum*," wrote Descartes, two centuries before Darwin —speaking truer than he knew. Were he alive today, he might well have changed that famous observation to "we think, therefore we have survived."

If I seem to belabor the point, it is for what seems to me a pressing reason. All too easily, we can agree that man can be called a learning animal and that he has a big brain. Having thus given lip service we utterly fail to act on the tremendous implications of man's nature.

We need to appreciate fully the degree of man's specialization as we probe into the human brain. Consider the elephant. Animals that live on the earth's surface are characteristically constructed so that they can bring their nose and mouth to ground level. They must do so to smell tracks or scent markers, usually to eat, and almost always to drink. It is no coincidence that the neck is long enough to permit reaching ground level. The elephant has developed an alternative solution: its neck is short but its trunk amply long. The proboscis can sniff a trail, suck in water, or gather food to be conveyed to the mouth.

The trunk is a highly specialized feature of the evolutionary "design" of this creature. Now let us ask a silly question: will the elephants use their trunks? Since it is apparent that the very existence of this species depends on trunk use, can we possibly conceive of a negative answer? True, instances can be found of design elements that hang on for many thousands of years after they have become obsolete (the main function of the appendix now seems to be to keep surgeons prosperous), but this is clearly due to nature's extreme conservatism, and the nonfunctional aspect of these residuals is usually apparent.

The human brain, looked at physically, parallels the elephant's trunk—it is a bizarre and freakish improbability, a wild excursion of nature, so out of keeping with the general order of life on this planet that an ingenious sophist could well construct a most impressive case proving it impossible. But to relate our brain adequately to the pachydermatous appendage, we would have to visualize an elephant with a trunk ten miles long. The brain is that odd, that preposterous.

Can we suppose that this astounding specialized feature is not used by the creatures that possess it? Can we assume that nature is so muddle-headed as to have given man this feature, but forgotten to provide motivation to use it?

The problem is less one of finding the answer to those questions than of explaining how people possessing this fabulous apparatus can fail to note the absurdities implicit in motivation. In fact, motivation serves as a broad cover-up word "used to account for" awkward gaps in knowledge or to gloss over the use of raw power to control other individuals.

Let us briefly trace this brain, this ten-mile-long trunk, further back in time.

If we define brain for the moment as a distinct, integrated agglomeration of nervous tissue having clearly dominant control over the organism, we have to note at the outset that the great majority of living creatures do not have brains. Of the more than one million species within the animal kingdom, only a few percent would qualify. To have a brain, any kind of brain, is to be exceptional.

While some invertebrates, including insects, have ganglionic brains (with various neuron systems in one "chamber," but not significantly integrated), true brains tend to be associated only with the phylum Chordata—one of the twenty-four phyla—and particularly with the subphylum Vertebrata, creatures with backbones. But other associations prove more significant. The first is that brain bears a strong connection to locomotion—at least in the negative sense that an organism that does not move around on its own a good deal is most unlikely to have much in the way of brain. (Extremely small organisms, of course, may simply not have the size and resources to devote a lot of cells to brain purposes, though they may move around incessantly.)

This relationship is understandable enough in terms of need. A shelled mollusk attached to a rock and feeding from passing currents will hardly benefit by having much brain. At the other extreme, an octopus moves around considerably, and has enormously more in the way of a nervous system. But the octopus does not move far and tends to remain in a limited, stable environment. The insects with larger "brains" are typically those that fly or crawl in exploratory fashion. Among vertebrates, brain power and the extent of locomotion tend to be highly correlated. As a creature adventures, it encounters a variety of conditions and circumstances in its search for sustenance or sexual activities. The decisions it has to make become more varied, numerous, and complex. To make a decision in the true sense of thinking requires taking in enough information through receptors to permit recognizing or classifying the situation, and then ordering a course of action.

The more alternative actions that can be taken, the harder the decision becomes—as such activities as shopping or selecting from a long menu remind humans. Choices between advance or retreat, fight or flee, run or hide, involving only a yes-or-no quality, have a simplicity that disappears when many actions and combinations of actions become available. Simultaneously, the importance of the decisions and the speed with which they must be made have bearing on the quality of brain needed.

If a creature has one standard kind of food that is plentiful all year round, it has minimal need of brain to obtain it. If its food supply shifts with the seasons, it needs more. If food often becomes scarce, and must be more widely searched for, the brain requirements rise again; if food must be stored to span shortage, still more. If the food supply consists of smaller organisms that can evade, we are likely to find further need for both brain power and alertness; and when the prey can not only escape but fight back in some way, another large jump in brain resources becomes indicated.

As we noted earlier, many apparently intelligent behaviors of insects, birds, and reptiles are built-in procedures that are merely triggered in some way and so set into action. The scent of a female can send a male moth on a seeking exploration, without anything we could call thinking—the moth has no choice, but must respond, exactly as a doorbell, if in working order, must respond in a fixed way when the button is pushed. For the insect that operates almost entirely on this basis a brain with neurons numbered in hundreds may suffice. But the mouse, which must perceive and respond to situations, and which lives in danger of becoming a meal everytime it seeks one, requires a brain with neurons counted in the millions.

We can feel fairly confident about many broad evolutionary aspects of man's long development. Far, far back, our line very likely took the form of quite small, defenseless animals, who survived largely by smell and alertness—fast decision making. Undoubtedly our forebears lived for long ages in trees, where needs favored selection of those with keen, stereoptic vision, brains able to control muscles with high accuracy and smoothness, hands and feet (and probably tails) that could grasp branches securely—and that developed far more delicacy and sensitivity than paws—and the opposed thumb to favor holding. Living in trees made errors uncomfortable (if not fatal) in just moving about, let alone avoiding enemies—high reliability had to be added to the inherited alertness.

For some good reason, probably climatic change, our line came down from the trees. Had we gone to the relative safety of dense forest, we might today be a species like monkey or gorilla. But savannahs or grasslands with little shelter became the habitat, at least for a long period; still more brain power was needed to scratch a living and stay alive. Bands had a better chance than individuals, and so social patterns, heavily dependent on brain, tended to develop. At some point, probably relatively late, social needs favored those who could communicate best, and speech appeared—an utterly new achievement for living creatures. The relation of speech to further brain development has chicken-and-egg aspects. Only an already impressive brain could utilize many sounds, and the utility of verbal communication clearly would favor those who had more than average brain power, and so could use communication to expanding purposes.

Ordinarily evolutionary developments tend to be self-limiting. For example, a long neck enables the giraffe to feed off high growth; but too long a neck would have diminishing utility and would increasingly become a handicap to fast running. Larger ears help a bat that flies by the guidance of a sonar system, but overly large ears would create too much air resistance. A working balance or trade-off has to be struck.

Man's brain, time may prove, is no exception. It could even now destroy us. It possibly could become so complex that it would fail to function properly too often to permit survival. But until now available evidence suggests that the trade-off point has not been reached. If it is advantageous to have huge brain power, man has been incredibly lucky—like a person who goes to a large county fair and wins prizes at every booth. Our development has been marked by a long succession of events and happenstances that were precisely those needed to encourage brain expansion. And so we are brain freaks. Chimpanzees and some other primates are brain freaks, too, but hardly in our class. In the evolutionary circus, we rate unquestionably as the star of the side show, but in our conceit we tend to think of ourselves as normal.

A well-endowed insect has perhaps a few thousand neurons; a dull vertebrate perhaps a thousand times as many, or some millions, to take a very rough base point. To get a brain on man's scale, we have to multiply those millions more than 10,000 times. The number of neurons in the human brain is usually estimated at ten to thirty billion or more, the estimates varying in part due to the technical approach. We need not quibble over the point: the numbers are stupefyingly large.[4] There are far more neurons in any one brain than there are people on earth. There are more possible interconnections between neurons in your brain, by manyfold, than between all the telephones that exist—they run into the trillions, to numbers beyond all ordinary meaning. To speak of the brain as comparable to an elephant's trunk ten miles long may be simple-minded and more colorful than scientific, but it does give the idea.

For those who like to play the game of comparing the human brain to computers, roughly equating neurons with diodes and transistors, it quickly becomes apparent than the natural apparatus puts the man-made to shame. A computer of the latest generation with anything like the capacity of an average brain would fill several large buildings and would require electric power sufficient to run a small city.

We humans are brain freaks. To suppose that we are endowed with this stupendous apparatus, but that we have to be motivated to use it, is to commit an absurdity magnificent in magnitude, but hardly for that reason admirable.

We do not need to urge children to use their brains. Our big task is to get out of their way. This masterpiece of creation is housed in bone armor and cushioned in fluid to protect it as much as possible from external shock; but it remains exceedingly vulnerable to input shocks from the very people who are supposed to be guarding the child's welfare—parents and teachers. The history and construction of the brain make inhibition of its proper and possible functions all too easy; and schools particularly have a devastating effect on millions of their charges. Conceived long ago in ignorance of how the brain works, these educational institutions contribute, I submit, to the generation or aggravation of anxiety, timidity, self-deprecation, and the kind of paranoidal citizenship|evidenced in everyday headlines.

Fortunately, change is under way, if far too slowly. Today almost no educators of any note will defend the old system, even though they suffer it to continue. Parents have become increasingly uneasy and less trusting of schools. The cry is for "humane" schools and a society that offers better personal living. Yet only as we begin to understand that brain that so dominates our unique nature among the millions of forms of life can we hope to achieve much progress in these directions.

CHAPTER 6

Not One Brain but Three

WHEN MAN'S fishy ancestors began to crawl out of the waters that incubated life and try their luck on the now cooler and more hospitable shore areas and then on dry land, they had problems. One was that their skins leaked. An outer covering that will serve well in water may be far from adequate to retain moisture when exposed to air and sun.[1] Amphibians had to develop better skins. The whole thrust of evolution up to this point was for living in the sea, an arrangement too complex to change. New skins provided the solution: they would permit the creatures to continue living in a saline fluid environment, but it would be internalized, carried around rather than being around.

In that sense we still live in the sea—in a fluid that in all likelihood has quite precisely the same salinity as the oceans of those far-off eons. Our tolerance for variation from the normal proportion of salt remains very small. We feel intense thirst if salinity gets too high and can suffer prostration if it gets too low. By various mechanisms our internal sea must be held within narrow limits.

In the same general way, higher forms of life developed the remarkable capacity, lacked by most species, to self-regulate body temperature; again, in all probability, basically to maintain temperatures common in those ancient seas. Our tolerance here, too, is small

—very little on the down side (unless induced), and only a few degrees above normal before acute symptoms result.

The arrangement for maintaining this kind of balance within limits is called homeostasis. In a broad sense, the human body consists of an enormously elaborate assortment of balancing or offsetting devices. The brain manages them.[2]

Perhaps the most familiar analogous mechanical device of this sort is the thermostat—for example, the one on the wall that controls a gas or oil furnace. If this device is set at 70 degrees, at about 68 it will signal "too cold" to the furnace and set it running. When the room heats up to around 72, it will send the message "hot enough" and the furnace will cut out. Such a homeostat is rather crude and merely sets limits within which the condition controlled oscillates. More sophisticated arrangements would provide continuous adjustment, as least under light load or stress, keeping the oscillations very small. Under severe load one way or the other, other systems might be called on for help. Electric power plants work this way; the generators constantly adjust to demand, up to a point at which other power sources must be cut in.

A thermostat in an electric iron deals with only heat as of the passing moment. The one on the wall, however, usually has a clock connected, that changes the setting, or *bias*, to perhaps 65 degrees at night, to economize on fuel. It is concerned with both heat and time. Obviously homeostats can become more and more complex as they monitor more and more factors. A fuel-injection system for an automobile engine may require a fairly elaborate little computer to "consider" all the factors affecting fuel requirements, such as engine temperature, air intake temperature, load, deceleration, acceleration. With these variables, a huge number of conditions become possible, and the fuel fed in must be exactly right to meet each need.

Not only have we a great many homeostatic systems monitoring a great many factors in the body, but they are frequently mutually responsive—what one does affects many others. We need quite a substantial amount of brain, then, to run these systems. We need more to change the biases, to adjust for some stress such as a fight or dangerous situation, or to destress as for rest or sleep.

The control of our muscles is also based on a push-pull arrangement. We extend an arm by relaxing one muscle and tightening another and retract it by the reverse procedure. This sounds simple, but to achieve delicate and precise control again requires a considerable amount of brain apparatus. Even the most limited actions involve many sets of muscles; they must be exactly balanced in push-pull to allow the movement to be started rapidly, slowed before the target is reached, and stopped without overshoot; and the force must be adjusted to the need—to pick up an egg, or to lift a 50-pound block. Much of the coordination called for is provided by the cerebellum, or "little brain" at the back of the brain, resting on the brain stem, where the spinal cord enters.

The cerebellum, a structure slightly smaller than a tennis ball, is concerned with execution. If we have never danced the polka but now attempt it, we will be clumsy and jerky—until the cerebellum learns to send a smooth flow of orders to all the scores of muscle sets involved. But the decision to polka must come from the cortex or outer layers of the brain. The visual perception that tells us where the floor is comes from the cortical center at the back of the brain, the aural perception of the music from another section, the kinesthetic perceptions that keep balance from yet another. Every second, hundreds of thousands of bits of information stream into the brain reporting where various muscles are, what stresses are on them, and what changes are in progress—plus reports on conditions in many other systems that must respond to the extra effort of trying to dance. This flood of simultaneous input to be analyzed, evaluated, and coordinated in "real time" (without appreciable delay) would bring the largest man-made computer to a gibbering breakdown from overload.

We can begin to see the pattern of evolutionary development. As man became a more complex being, his nervous systems had to elaborate in proportion; the two aspects of complexity had to grow hand in hand. Our brain was never "designed" in the sense that an architect designs a house or an engineer a machine. Little by little, over many millions upon millions of years, it grew more complex in response to need. To leave the sea and in time become an amphibious form required new systems and new brain resources to manage them; to become a land animal able to maintain a set body temperature (unlike insects and reptiles that must slow activity as temperature falls) demanded still more. To come down from the trees much later on and risk open country created new needs; to use tools and words and to hunt dangerous game added again and again to physical and brain complexity.

But the brain was never "rationalized," never modernized. Like the country house, built over many years, where the new color television sits on part of the original foundation wall, the brain is a hodgepodge of parts of varying antiquity, reflecting its origins. That even some of the most insightful experimental psychologists have tended to ignore this plain fact must be counted an instance of the fragmentation that characterizes the field.[3]

It is tempting to try to separate brain functions into those that regulate processes inside our organism and those that deal with the environment outside. For some limited uses, this may prove convenient. But in general any such division sets us off on a wrong track right away.

Far back, our line had a fishlike form. To emerge on land, our precursors had to evolve legs from fins or paddles. It plainly is rather foolish to look at such legs as being "inside," since they make no sense except as response to environment. The only way we can separate from our environment is to die, and even that could be argued. Both in terms of physical structure and nervous apparatus, our evolutionary development simply holds a mirror to our environment. Nor does nature forget readily. If it has developed a leg from a fin, it continues to follow essentially the same route to produce a leg long after. It may telescope the process to a degree, but it has no way of abruptly introducing a new way to get a leg—as a human designer could. The intricate bones of our ears are conversions of those that once supported gills when we swam in the ocean.[4] The cells that form sperm or ova are remakes of what long before composed a now discarded egg sac.

This principle must be noted as one of fundamental importance. Because of the way evolution operates, the design of a species is always built on what went before. There can be amplification, modification, reapplication, and (rarely) simplification. There can be mutation—an accidental change in genes that is passed on to succeeding generations. Mutations, however, occur very seldom. (In J. J. Muller's well-known study with the fruit fly *Drosophila*, 400 were detected in 20 million subjects.) The great bulk of mutations do not have lasting effect, and those that do succeed will usually make only an extremely small change in the organism, leaving the rest unaffected. No mechanism exists to enable radical change to occur quickly, nor to allow "quantum jumps," nor to introduce major new arrangements. Even the process of shedding the obsolete and useless can take millions of years, as a glance at the nipples on a male chest reminds us. This principle pervades nature. It would be astonishing if it were not reflected in the basic nature of the human brain.

Anyone who has bred domestic animals selectively understands that there is no way to "make something out of nothing." If a trait or characteristic exists in a parent, possibly it can be accentuated by selective breeding over many generations—a deliberate and only occasionally successful hurrying-up of the usual evolutionary processes for narrow purposes. No way exists to breed a green cow, unless some trace of suitable genes can be found in living cows. What has gone before must be the foundation.

To grasp the significance of the structure of the human brain, we must trace it far back in time. For brevity, we can begin with the image of a spinal cord, extending down the back of a bilaterally symmetrical creature, contrasting with the numerous other nervous system arrangements, in much wider use throughout the animal kingdom. In vertebrates this all-important gathering of nerve tissue is protected by bone much as the brain is. It runs right through the spinal column.

A bilaterally symmetrical creature has a front and a rear. It locomotes in one direction (although it may be able to back up if necessary), and consequently the front end far more frequently encounters changes in its environment. Understandably, the increase in nervous tissue needed to deal with changes occurs at the front end, convenient to such organs as mouth, tongue, nose, eyes, feelers, heat sensors, or ears. A *head* is the result—a feature most living creatures don't have.

If indeed brain control could easily divide into inside and outside parameters, we would expect to find two brains, one at the head end for responding to the environment, and one probably centrally located for internal affairs. Some ganglia, or small aggregations, do occur in various parts of the body; the solar plexus has gained some fame as a target in boxing, although it is not located where commonly supposed, but higher up and behind the stomach. In creatures having much simpler nervous systems than man, these subbrains may have a larger role; but because in man inside and outside cannot very well be separated, the brain in the head runs the whole show.

In all probability the brain began developing as an enlargement at the head of a primitive spinal cord, which early on took the form of a tube.[5] (The brain has internal spaces called ventricles and so is still a tube, though much distorted.) The swelling was not uniform, but rather produced three "bumps," mostly on the top, as Figure 1 suggests.

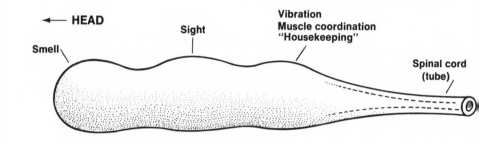

Figure 1

The front swelling was required to deal with olfactory inputs, for smell was the earliest sensitive receptor to develop able to discern the environment at a distance. The midsection thickened to provide more neurons that could handle inputs from light detection or vision; this specialized sensitivity was at first probably located at the top of the body and only crudely responsive to light and warmth from the sun. Only later did it become still more specialized into eyes. The hind section, from which eventually arose the cerebellum, was nearest to the muscles it controlled for motion, balance, vibration detection, and also much of the routine "housekeeping" apparatus of blood circulation, oxygen supply, digestion, and other such internal systems that required more central brain direction as they became increasingly complex.

Although this pattern was developing somewhere around a half-billion years ago, we should not think of it as ancient history. The consequences affect us now.

The function of this early brain, overall, was to receive information, process it, and reach decisions expressed ultimately in behavior —which still remains the brain's main task. But input in two or more modes had to be compared. An attractive odor might indicate "go" while a threatening shadow signaled "flee." Or, an olfactory input might signify "food probable in this area" if moving objects of a certain size were seen. Cross-modal comparison and evaluation was essential to interpret input and reach a decision. In short, the different parts of the brain might heartily agree, or argue, or produce confusingly contradictory reports.

For a time, apparently, the midsection that handled vision was in the driver's seat, and this still appears true in fish and amphibia. But as our line moved out onto land and mammals evolved, scent assumed greater importance. What C. U. M. Smith refers to in *The Brain* as "the head office" moved to the front section. He notes:

> It seems probable that olfaction is the dominant sense in many mammalian groups. Hunting, socializing, mating, escaping—all depend to a greater or lesser extent on olfactory cues and clues. The perceptual worlds of most mammals are predominantly olfactory worlds.[6]

Any dog owner can attest to this observation. He may say he takes his pet out for a walk, but as far as the dog is concerned, the outing is for a smell. The animal will sniff, and leave (if male) scent markers to other sniffers who may follow. For man, having lost much of this typically mammalian receptivity, the dog's behavior retains a bizarre quality no matter how familiar it may become. It is not easy to get into another creature's modalities.

From these swellings on the front end of the spinal cord to man's present brain extends a long and progressively more complex path. The point for the moment must be that it is a path, a totally continuous development in which the new was, in general, added to the old, primitive centers. These remain, their functions modified to a degree, but still very much present, still functional, still playing essential roles in determining behavior. Unless we view the human brain in this light, we can never really make sense of it.

In evolutionary terms, we do not have *a* brain, but a group of brains—three, for convenience of discussion—of very different antiquity and powers. The relationships among these brains, and their interactions, are of the utmost importance.

CHAPTER 7

Something New in Gray Matter

THIS BOOK is not about the brain, but rather about how the brain functions to make us behave and learn in certain ways. For the purpose of constructing Proster Theory, we do not have to go very deeply into the brain's neurophysiology, so long as the broad outlines we draw are firmly based on the present large and well-established body of knowledge. We do need, however, to explore the three-brain aspect of the apparatus enough to understand its general architecture.

The three enlargements of the early nerve chord had fairly specific main assignments: that in the front dealt with smell, the middle section with light, the posterior one with vibration, internal systems, and muscle coordination. As always in discussing biological matters, we need to beware of simplifications: smell and light and vibration cover a lot of ground. In the beginning these brain centers were essentially receptors, sensitive to certain aspects of the environment. With time and evolution, they became far more sensitive and broader in range.

It may be helpful at this point to consider complexity of input. A vast amount of behavior in lower level animals lies close to what we can call "simple circuit." Push the button, and the doorbell rings —it must ring, assuming the circuit is intact. Among reptiles, fish, and birds, this simple circuit, which so readily translates into the conventional stimulus-response of the psychologist, plays a great part, producing what seem to be much more intelligent actions. For example, ethologist Niko Tinbergen showed that the newly hatched herring gull pecks at its parent's bill because it has a red spot near the end.[1] The spot is like the doorbell button. Wooden or cardboard objects of various shapes with a red spot will trigger the pecking, objects lacking the red spot won't. The chick is born with this simple circuit built in.

In the same fashion, the newly hatched cuckoo pushes the eggs of the rightful owners of the nest out to destruction, so it will get all the food. The mechanism is simple circuit; the cuckoo hatches earlier, and for a few days has a built-in drive to push when a sensitive spot on its body contacts an object. No thought is involved. I recall a striking photograph of a warbler feeding a cuckoo chick, so much bigger than the poor host that the warbler has to stand on the cuckoo's head to drop insects into its gaping mouth. But the warbler has no alternative. Its built-in simple circuits require it to feed any red open mouth in its nest.

Suppose you have a job in an office. When the phone on your desk rings, you are required to answer it. This is a simple circuit, though a voluntary one: you have the power to refuse should you so decide. Now assume an intercom is installed with another phone, which you are to answer if a light comes on. You now have two separate simple circuits, which lead to similar actions of picking up one phone or the other.

Let us add more complexity. The system is changed. The intercom is also given a ring. The outside phone rings in this pattern:

RINGGGGGG   (Pause)   RINGGGGG   (Pause)   RINGGGGG

The intercom has a different ring:

RING–RING–RING   (Pause)   RING–RING–RING   (Pause)

Now the simple circuit has been left behind. To determine which phone to pick up, you have to identify one pattern rather than another. The doorbell kind of stimulus no longer applies. The simple circuit can't distinguish patterns—a much more complicated device would be needed to accomplish that.[2]

Let us say now that you are instructed to answer the outside phone anytime, but the intercom ring only if the light comes on. This means that in addition to detecting patterns of ring, you have to use two modes—sound and light—to make your action decision. What if the light comes on but the intercom doesn't ring? You then have cross-modal conflict, or conflicting input. What do you do? Either you do nothing, or you "call the boss"—somehow refer the conflict to higher authority for resolution.

Add one more level of complexity. You are told to answer the intercom regardless of the light between noon and one o'clock, and not to answer the other phone after five. Now you must deal with sound, sight, and time to make any action decision. You not only have to determine pattern but also situation. You accept the stimulus of the light under some conditions but not under others—which begins to make the entire stimulus concept pretty confusing. Inhibition—don't answer under certain conditions—becomes an offset to stimulus, reminding us of the homeostats we have discussed.

Even this brief excursion into thinking indicates how rapidly complexity can build up. To cope with it, the brain must provide increasing amounts of "gray matter"—neurons capable of effecting decisions (in contrast to "white matter," or tissues which conduct nerve messages from one place to another). Our spinal cord, which with the brain composes the central nervous system, consists largely of white tissue carrying information to or from the brain, but a certain amount of gray matter is also distributed throughout the column, to influence the flow of information. The great bulk of gray matter is in the brain.

How can neurons make decisions? We need not regard this as too miraculous. We have frequent occasion to insert a key in a lock. If the key fits the tumblers and the lock's stops, it can turn, withdraw the bolt, and admit us. If the key does not match, the lock decides not to admit us. We may not commonly think of this as a decision, but clearly it is. A coin-operated vending machine may be a bit more complex. Its apparatus considers the size and weight of the coin, its thickness, and its magnetic qualities before deciding that the coin is genuine, and, if so, disgorges the product. Otherwise it bypasses the coin to a slot as a reject. The machine plainly decides what to do on the basis of the inputs it receives. But even this mechanical device is not just passive. It actively tests the coin for the qualities it demands.

There seems little reason to get into mystical areas in dealing with brain, rather than regarding it as apparatus. Experimenters have built electronically controlled artificial animals that appear startlingly live in behavior.[3] As computers continue to develop, their ability to show "thinking" and "creative" behavior has markedly increased. To many people the idea that there is no sharp, firm boundary between apparatus or mechanisms and mind seems shocking and repulsive: it is taken as demeaning or even destroying the very human qualities we hold most precious.

But this seems, on analysis, mainly a matter of words. We think of machines as being simple, insensitive, and uncommunicative, so being compared to mechanisms, or told we are mechanisms, seems most insulting and degrading. But when we see a very intricate machine that is not limited to obvious repetitive actions, we are apt to say "it's almost human!" The remark is significant. It can lead us to suspect that what we see as human is essentially *complexity* and *sensitivity*—and the human brain is the most complex and multi-sensitive apparatus in our universe.[4]

A couple of hundred million years ago, however, the brain was merely the primitive tube with three swellings that we looked at in the last chapter. Let us return to it and briefly note what happened to it, particularly to its front end. As Figure 2 shows, the anterior portion, concerned with smell, divided into two lobes. The early gray matter was inside, encircling the open part or ventricle of the tube. But over a long period, in response to the need for more brain, this type of gray matter was pushed into the middle or down to the bottom to make room for something new: a much superior kind of gray matter, the neocortex, which moved to the outside (cortex means bark) where it would have more room—which the folding also aided. The cross section (B) suggests how the new kind of neurons began to take over.

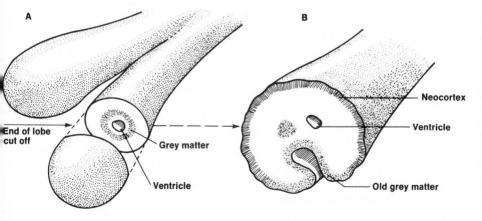

Figure 2

But this was only the beginning. The early gray matter had largely specific functions relating to smell or sight or some other modality. But the neocortex had the capability to integrate. It received information from the various receptor areas of the tube brain, and became the decision maker.

For analogy, we can think of a business that has a production department, a shipping room, a sales office, and an accounting section. The managers run their departments, consulting with each other only when necessary. The business could operate this way up to a point, but with increasing complexity the need for management would become more and more acute. A general manager, not linked to any one department, would be essential to make decisions and coordinate, based on information received from all departments. The neocortex became the general manager of the brain—but the old department heads stayed at their jobs.

In contrast to development in creatures such as insects that had ganglia in various places rather than a continuous tube, and no general manager (insects, as noted, have brains only in the sense that some ganglia are crowded into the head), the stage was now set for as much expansion of the manager's office as need might require.

We must appreciate here that there is no point in having more sensory input from the environment than can be interpreted, any more than in having ten telephone trunk lines feed into an office where there is only one phone. But the older gray matter was severely limited in its ability to interpret beyond very crude limits. The neocortex could handle far more detail. Thus over millions of years the new kind of gray matter took on more and more work of this kind, as well as integrating and making decisions; doing so gave the creature a survival advantage. In man, this meant a ballooning of the neocortex into our present cerebral hemispheres, with thousands of times more cortical surface. The middle swelling, which had been concerned with sight, lost most of this function to the new cortex, although input from the eyes still is routed through it. The rear swelling retained its regulatory duties, though under some control of the neocortex, and developed a much improved cerebellum or "little brain" at the rear, a marvelously compact and complex computer to better coordinate and direct muscular activity.

As it ballooned, the new brain formed a thick cap which almost surrounds and sits on the moderately developed midbrain and hindbrain. In no other creature has the forebrain developed to anything approaching this extent; this is the distinguishing physical mark that so sharply sets off man from all other animals. Mammals in general show this mushrooming of the forebrain, but even the large apes, who come closest, are scarcely serious rivals. The rat's neocortex compares to ours roughly as a pea does to a watermelon.

Figure 3 shows in simplified form the human brain looked at from below, so the relatively enormous size of the "cap" can be appreciated. Yet we must bear in mind that it's not something really new, or extra, but only a development to extreme degree of the same neural tube that led to all true brains. It is still very much part of the tube, intricately tied in with the rest of the brain.

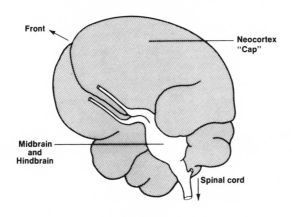

Figure 3

The original structure can be traced back stage by stage (and also embryonically)—fortunately, because otherwise the brain plan might seem quite mad. The eyes, for example, now by far the most important receptors for man, are in the front of the head, connected to the midbrain, and yet the data received is synthesized in the rearmost portion of the cortex, the occipital lobes.

It should be stated, of course, that the brain is laterally quite symmetrical, with the two cerebral hemispheres roughly, but by no means exactly, mirror images. The surface is heavily convoluted, a process that began very long ago, perhaps to create more surface area or for other structural reasons. The size of the skull has limits set by the problems of birth, female locomotion, maturing period, minimum brain requirements at birth, and ultimate brain needs—an elaborate trade-off.

In function, the hemispheres are decidedly not mirror images. In most people, the control of speech occupies a large amount of the left-side lobes, attesting to the enormous importance of verbal abilities to humans. Part of the right side usually handles visual-spatial relations, the mapping we need to relate to our environment and to find our way around. Obviously this need goes back further than speech. Music and some aspects of mathematics are also normally right-side activities.

The two sides of the cortical brain, however, are connected by a large crossover, the *corpus callosum*. Experiments have been conducted on animals in which the halves are surgically separated (some cases exist in humans), in effect producing double-brained subjects who do not transfer what is learned from one side to the other.[5] In the normal brain, the two sides are fully coordinated. In fact it is not too much to say as a generality that every part of the brain is connected with every other part—a reason why unravelling its detailed plan has been so difficult. With the partial exception of one central strip of motor-control areas related to specific portions of the body, the brain tends to be diffuse and highly redundant—very far from the telephone switchboard it was commonly described as a generation or two ago.

Quite astonishingly large amounts of brain tissue can be destroyed or cut out of the cortex without producing a great deal of obvious change in physical behavior, especially if a recovery period is allowed. The most famous case involves an explosives foreman named Phineas Gage, who by accident had a thick steel tamping rod driven through the front of his skull. By one account, the unfortunate Mr. Gage did not even faint. He lived for many years after, suffering personality changes, but actively carrying on his own affairs.[6]

A way of looking at our three brains that is more meaningful for our present purposes than hindbrain, midbrain, and forebrain has been provided by Dr. Paul D. MacLean of the National Institute of Mental Health, a very prominent brain researcher. He calls the oldest and innermost the "reptilian" brain. It comprises the brain stem, part of the midbrain, and some other structures plus a rudimentary cortex. Surrounding this is the "old mammalian" brain, which includes what is called the limbic system. Capping this in turn is the neocortex, or "new mammalian" brain. Figure 4 (after MacLean) suggests this concept.

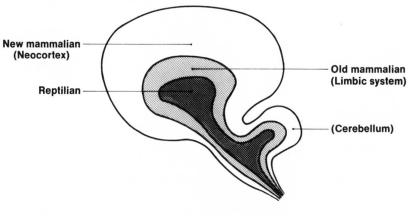

New mammalian
(Neocortex)

Reptilian

Old mammalian
(Limbic system)

(Cerebellum)

Figure 4

These are suggestive and useful terms for Proster Theory. As we shall see, the triple nature of our brains has a most important bearing on how we learn.

Our reptilian brain largely reflects a moderate improvement of the brains creatures had roughly three hundred million years ago as they emerged from the waters to try their luck on land. In water, a quite limited degree of smell, sight, and vibration detection served adequately to find food and mates, and to avoid predators and dangers enough to allow the species to survive and perpetuate itself. Decisions could be made mainly on the basis of species wisdom— behaving in set patterns, often by what I have called doorbell or simple circuits. Certain smells, for example, meant "food, get it," others "danger, swim away," and so on. Discrimination could be crude, decisions fairly uncomplicated. Gray matter was needed to sort out these inputs, coordinate across modalities, and make decisions—but not much, by later standards. Individual learning was meager.

On land, demands increased even for reptiles. Conditions varied more, temperatures rose and fell, gravity had greater effect, locomotion had to adjust to a variable terrain. But while more gray matter was needed, the old plan still held.

We find this kind of brain the entire brain in existing reptiles, and in our own heads as the oldest of our three brains. We should not despise our human, improved version of it too quickly; it is still a most impressive brain compared to those of the vast majority of creatures belonging to that elite who have brains at all. It does a remarkable job of managing our many body homeostats that control salinity, sugar levels, body temperature, capillaries and blood pressure, and a long list of other functions that used to be called involuntary but are no longer so glibly termed. It not only sends messages by nerves (like telegraphed orders) but also by influencing the addition of hormones to the blood (like broadcast orders). And that superb miniaturized computer, the cerebellum, brilliantly coordinates the more than 600 muscle structures of the body for such complex tasks as reading, riding a bicycle, playing a violin, or keeping balance while running across rough ground in a high wind.

Our middle or "old mammalian" brain, in MacLean's terminology, reflects that stage of our development when our ancestors were small mammals, surviving by being far more alert, sensitive to conditions, and quick in response than the reptilian types from which man branched off. Such creatures had to be far more aware of situation, and have far more available programs—not only fixed species wisdom, but new, currently useful, individually and perhaps socially learned tactics. Even the homeostats, now grown more elaborate in order to provide faster and more varied responses to emergencies, had to be subject to greater range of bias, to be able to apply greater resources to a short, quick effort of attack or escape adapted to the situation.

Not at all surprisingly, then, we find that this middle brain has a considerable cortex of gray matter, as well as some other centers within its mass; and we also find here the limbic area greatly concerned with what we call emotions—which will be discussed in the next chapter.

Capping this brain is the preposterously developed new mammalian brain, with its relatively huge sheet of gray matter, the cerebral neocortex. All mammals possess it, but none in such quantity as some primates, and no primate in such magnificence as man. Compared to older gray matter, it is enormously more complex and capable. This cortex is what we think of when we speak generally of the powers of the human brain—but we must remember that it does not exist in isolation. It is linked, as recent neurological research has shown more and more in a variety of investigations, to the earlier mammalian brain, and to the much earlier reptilian brain. The learning and behavior effected by the brain as a whole cannot be understood—no more than we can understand "face" unless we juxtapose eyes, nose, and mouth—except as we consider the interactions.

MacLean's picture of the three-brains-in-one reflects his strong evolutionary orientation. It will be helpful here to consider briefly a different but compatible concept, that of the Soviet scientist A. R. Luria. Investigating from a psychoneurological approach, heavily based on studies of impairment due to lesions or wounds (particularly those suffered by Soviet soldiers during World War II), Luria emphasizes function. He too sees the brain in terms of three "blocks."

His first block takes in the brain stem and is concerned with "energy level" and "tone" of the cortex, a central portion of which is directly involved. It functions as a sort of primary mechanism in our present, modern brains, concerned with wakefulness, alertness, and with organizing brain processes in general.

Luria's second block is chiefly concerned with the reception, analysis, and storage of information. Occupying the rear portion of the cortex, it is as specific as the first block is general; and instead of neurons mingling in a network, they here become functionally isolated. Many have single-sense jobs: sight only, or sound only, for example; others are multimodal.

The third block comprises the frontal lobes and has no sensory, perception, speech or motor functions, but is concerned with, in Luria's words, "the formation of intentions and programs for behavior."[7] This, then, is on the basis of very substantial evidence, today's head office.

Luria sees the second block as in itself having three levels of organization and function. The first receives the sensory, single-mode inputs ("projection" areas, in Luria's terms), the second level (projection-association) relates one mode to another, and the third (zones of overlapping) performs a synthesis of incoming and stored information. The three levels are progressively more sophisticated and complex.

Brain researchers, of whatever discipline, solidly agree that as the brain has developed, the tendency has been for the newer portions not to replace but to elaborate the earlier functions—somewhat as a person might obtain a very simple hand-size transistor radio, then progress to a more sensitive and powerful AM/FM table model with more controls, and eventually to a monstrous high-fidelity system, stereo and quadraphonic with many functions and peripherals . . . all the time retaining and continuing to use the earlier equipment.

But the researchers also agree that the brains, old and new, are permanently and intricately "wired together." It can be helpful to speak of three brains or three blocks, but we should always remember to add "in one."

Though terrifyingly complex, the human brain is a single, indivisible apparatus in its functions. This now evident fact helps explain why the long efforts of many psychologists to understand behavior by experimental fragments have so consistently produced less than satisfactory answers.

CHAPTER 8

Switches, Biasing, Emotions

What we are seeking to build in this discussion is a model of how the human brain operates. The model will serve only if the concepts it involves are clear and well understood. It seems advisable, then, to discuss them one by one.

Consider the concept of switching.

A freight train stands loaded on a side track in a valley in California. It must reach a siding by a warehouse near Baltimore, three thousand miles away. To route it there sounds difficult, for hundreds of tracks crisscross the intervening territory; yet we can set forth in one brief instruction all that is required: each time the train comes to a switch, set that switch to take the train toward the warehouse in Baltimore. We can assume that at each switch there will be someone who will know which way to throw the switch, left or right. (There will always be a choice, if there is a switch, and never more than two options, so we are dealing with a binary system, such as digital computers use.)

Unless we are used to the idea, it is not easy to see this simple idea of a switch as having much to do with thinking, which we are apt to conceive of as mysterious, complicated, and exotic. In our daily experience, we deal with switches one at a time. Only when we have a lot of switches and can use them in sequences do we acquire the potentials that electronic computers illustrate. And our attention is usually not on the switch but on what results. We flip the switch on the wall to illuminate the room, or we turn the ignition key in the car to start the engine—it takes some effort to focus on the switch itself and see that moving it from open to closed, from off to on, expresses a decision.

A doorbell is a switch. Pressing the button closes a gap, completing the electric circuit and causing the bell to ring. The cuckoo chick has a sensitive spot on its chest, in effect a doorbell button. Touching it against an object closes the switch, causing the bird to push against the object, which normally would be one of the other, unhatched eggs. Similarly, the red spot on the beak of the herring gull is a visual switch that closes the circuit that produces pecking.

Recall the office situation we considered in the previous chapter, and translate it into switches (Figure 5a). With one phone we have the following:

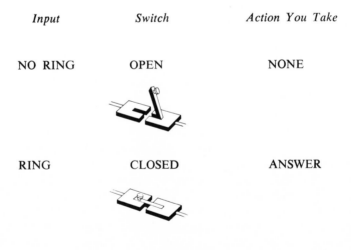

Input	*Switch*	*Action You Take*
NO RING	OPEN	NONE
RING	CLOSED	ANSWER

Figure 5a

Later in our example you were required to answer the main phone until five o'clock, but not after five. This can be set up in switch terms (Figure 5b) that show us sequence coming into play as follows:

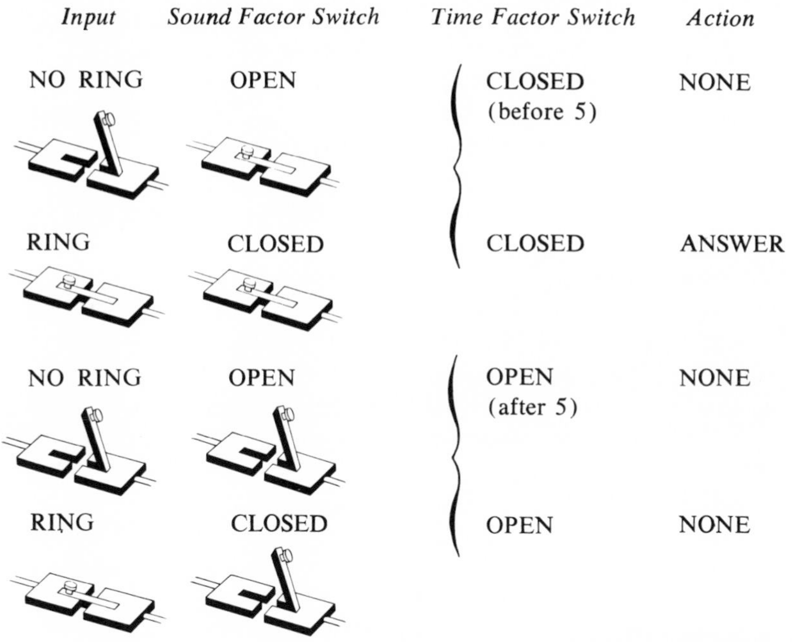

Input	Sound Factor Switch	Time Factor Switch	Action
NO RING	OPEN	CLOSED (before 5)	NONE
RING	CLOSED	CLOSED	ANSWER
NO RING	OPEN	OPEN (after 5)	NONE
RING	CLOSED	OPEN	NONE

Figure 5b

In computer terms, this would be an *and* circuit, because only when the sound switch and the time switch are closed will action follow. In computers, of course, the switches (diodes and transistors) physically exist. In the brain, they physically are present in vast numbers in the form of various kinds of neurons, special cells that exist only within the nervous system. In the cerebral cortex of the human brain well over twenty-five billion of these intricate cells are tightly packed, but as recent research has begun to show, they form a fairly orderly arrangement of columns (perpendicular to the surface of the cortex) and layers or levels (parallel to the cortical surface).

Most typically, a neuron has many input feeders entering the main portion or cell body, and an axon or output that leads from the cell body, in some cases extending several feet—if going, for example, to a muscle. The end of the axon is usually branched. Most neurons connect to other neurons via extremely small gaps called synapses, and the number of branches at each end can be large. Neurons that connect to other neurons within the central nervous system are called internuncial or interneurons, and may have very short axons, heavily branched at the end.

A great deal more is known now about how neurons work than was the case twenty years ago, and the investigations that extended this knowledge surely must rank among the most fascinating imaginable. Since the function of Proster Theory initially is to produce a simple model, we shall not go much further into technical aspects of neurons. It will serve our purpose to visualize brain operation in terms of switches and switching; and it becomes unimportant whether some aspects of switching are achieved by a single neuron or by neurons working in groups.

Much evidence suggests that inhibition is a more common function of neuronal switching than activation. The neuron is an electrochemical device, producing clearly detectable and measurable electric potentials and currents—including the "brain waves" recorded by the electroencephalograph, or EEG machine. These can be picked up by electrodes applied at various points on the head, so showing patterns of activation.

If you live in a house or a large apartment, chances are that at any time of day or night most of the electric outlets are ordinarily not in use. Many of the lamps and motors and heaters are off; we could say that with their switches being open, they are inhibited. Similarly, in the brain most of the almost infinite number of possible circuits are off. Even so, the brain when awake demands a greedy share of the body's energy supply: though weighing about one-fiftieth of the body total, it may use as much as one fifth of all the energy that is being consumed. The inhibitory system both prevents overloading and in many uses sharpens perceptions or information processing. Epilepsy, a fairly common brain condition, involves a small segment of the brain that for reasons not fully understood gets overactive and out of control, upsetting surrounding circuits to a greater or lesser degree. A seizure can cause anything from a brief interruption of normal functioning, hardly observable, to the *grand mal* fit that can produce unconsciousness and writhing for a period of some minutes. Such attacks suggest the hazards of overloading, but we do not have to worry that overloading by thinking will produce epilepsy. The capactiy of the human brain is so vast that in ordinary daily functioning we are hardly likely to employ more than a small fraction of its capabilities.

Since the reader has been promised that we will be considering more humane ways of educating children and dealing with people, it may seem that talking of brain switches is a strangely mechanistic way to that goal. We are about to look at emotions in the same evolutionary and mechanistic way. But we run no risk of demeaning man by realistically examining his amazing brain. On the other hand, we can frustrate ourselves by accepting and acting on distorted concepts of its nature. However odd it may seem, what some may call mechanistic approaches will get us faster and more surely to the humane goal than less austere and at first blush more direct pathways.

In normal health, emotions arise in the brain and nowhere else. Language is full of phrases that suggest a sharp dichotomy: "use your head, not your heart," "cognitive or affective," "rational, logical thinking, not gut reaction." Among educators who deal directly with children we can often detect, in those who lay stress on the child's "affective needs," a very strong tendency to speak as though the brain were concerned only with logic and intellectual pursuits, while the hands paint or sculpt or nurture animals or make music; and there are others who believe as deeply that physical contact, the laying on of hands, and the warm interactions of a functional group have a magic distinctly separate from thinking. This kind of separation of what are all brain concerns expresses, of course, a gross misconception of what thinking is. One may hazard the guess that the growing use of the computer, that hairless, skinless monster, has added to the dichotomy's power. To most people, a computer performs complex mathematical operations, the essence of logical thought (they forget that it does so essentially by very rapidly counting on its fingers and toes), and therefore accentuates the contrast between warm, affective basket weaving and cold calculating of sines, cosines, and tangents by mysterious and unhuman rituals.

This muddled view of brain functions strongly interferes with our achieving a unified theory of learning or human behavior.

We have already discussed the essential mechanisms of emotions: homeostats and bias. Visualize us as we saunter across a field, noting the wildflowers. Now we hear a sound and become aware of an approaching, apparently ill-disposed bull. We react to the threat of harm by an abrupt shift of bias. The settings of the homeostats are, so to speak, moved over to "emergency." Hormones pour into the blood, broadcasting alarms throughout the body—much as a siren system aboard a warship summons all hands to battle stations and conditions. The capillaries tighten, sending blood pressure up, while breathing and heartbeat change to allow maximum short-term effort. Some digestive processes stop or slow down. At length we reach a fence and scramble over. We now find that our legs feel as if they will buckle, our stomach as if someone has tied knots in it, and our hand shakes as with palsy. It takes some time before the hormones' effects subside and the biases reset to their customary levels.

This emergency shift of bias lies at the core of what we call emotion; and overwhelming evidence shows that the shift is controlled in and by the brain.[1] We had to interpret the situation of being in the field with the bull as threatening—purely a thinking process—and as a consequence throw the switches that set us running for the fence and released hormones to permit maximum short-term effort. It is worth noting that the "master gland" of the intricate endocrine system is the pituitary, which grows directly from the base of the brain—from the back portion of what was the frontmost of the three lobes. This makes sense in evolutionary terms, since this was the olfactory center, and smell was originally the dominant distant receptor. The panic button was located conveniently close to where the panic warning came in.

Emotions or emergency biasing became more complex just as brain operations did, and by parallel development. For a fish not able to put up a defense, the prime emotional response was to flee. If it had some morphological weapon such as teeth to permit attack, it had the option to flee or fight—a choice requiring an evaluation of the situation in order to throw the right switch. On land, an agile small mammal could escape by a variety of tactics: freezing or playing dead, running away at top speed, evasive turning, entering a burrow, or climbing a tree. More choices mean more switches, which in turn mean more gray matter to make decisions after evaluating the situation. The hormone combinations needed to freeze or to dart into a burrow and remain silent differ from those needed for a ten-minute run. More patterns of biasing, more bias switches, are required—which involves development of more emotional capabilities.

Initially emotions were directly related to survival needs—and some still are. Failure to escape meant death, a meal for a predator. For the attacker, failure to win the fight meant losing a meal and if food was scarce, possible starvation. But as situations became more complex and choices multiplied, less intense emotions developed. Ordinarily a predator does not attack a potential victim unless it believes, by experience or species wisdom, that it will win. If the odds seem too even, the confrontation may end in a standoff. So it can be useful for the intended victim to give signals of willingness to fight. This calls for a bias less extreme than that required for full flight or attack. A further step down may be appropriate for more distant meetings—a readying that signals "stay out of my way" or "avoid me and I'll avoid you." Biasing by hormones produces very convincing and easily read signals, such as the arched back of a cat, the expanded fur of many animals, or the posture produced by tensed muscles.

As we come to social animals, the need for signals greatly increases, and the range of biasing extends by many steps from enough to indicate minor annoyance, through disciplinary threat, to readiness to engage in deadly combat. In sexual matters, a bias of a kind not otherwise used may take control, setting off often elaborate rituals and behaviors that give powerful signals to rivals or to the opposite sex. In *The Mind of Man* Nigel Calder notes:

> Emotions are not feelings supplied gratuitously by nature; they serve very practical purposes, for aiding appropriate reactions to events and to other individuals, and for eliciting responses from others.[2]

The essential point is that emotions and signals are strongly and probably inseparably linked because of their evolutionary origins and functions.[3] This means that, in general if not always, one cannot give a signal to other humans without first producing the actual, physical, hormonal bias, and cannot produce the bias without to some degree giving the signal. We become rather expert, of course, in "smoke screening" signals we do not wish to send out by using behavioral devices and distractions, and verbalizations that conceal or distort. But I suspect that the successful gambler, while sharpening his ability to read genuine signals, also learns to control and forestall his own biasing—that is, not to let the emotion occur, not to let the hormones flow.

Ideas on the ability of the "conscious mind" to control what used to be considered involuntary functions have changed radically in recent years. Evidence has mounted that ordinary citizens can learn to modify their own blood pressure, for example, or even their brain waves. The long-rumored powers of oriental mystics and holy men over their bodies has been at least in large part authenticated. In *The Mind of Man* Calder reports in detail on a 1970 experiment with Ramanand Yogi as the subject, enclosed in an airtight box, closely monitored by complex apparatus which showed he could reduce his oxygen needs far below the supposed minimum required to survive. The dictionaries that define the autonomic system as "independent of will" appear to need some revisions.[4]

We have all had the experience, in many kinds of social or business situations, of sensing messages that are nonverbal or even counterverbal. "I enjoyed every minute," or "I'll try to help you in some way" is what a tape recorder would hear—but the signal comes across quite differently. Children in a classroom appear to have extraordinary ability to pick up nonverbal signals from teachers. As we shall see, such signals and the emotions they represent have, if Proster Theory is correct, enormous implications for encouraging or inhibiting learning.

Great progress has been made in recent years in mapping the emotional centers of the brain. Two main approaches serve to locate these centers. One is via epileptic attacks. Typically, a seizure is preceded by a warning or "aura," and the patient is able in many cases to note and report the consistent feeling experienced, which may be of great joy or elation, or deep dread or depression, or almost anything in between. In some instances, even experiencing a particular emotion may trigger an attack. Severe epilepsy in a relatively few cases is treated surgically, by removing the small portion of the brain that seems to be causing the trouble. Thus surgeons have important reason to compare the reported aura with specific locations in the brain. Electric probing often is performed before any excision. The brain itself has no pain receptors so it feels no pain when operated on. The patient can be fully conscious and able to report the results of the probing, which may produce emotions, memories, hallucinations, or muscle movements (or nothing at all) according to the location of the probe.

The second method involves systematic experimental probing of the brains of animals, in whom at least the grosser emotional reactions can be readily noted. Since probes can now be positioned with exquisite accuracy, much has been learned about the complex homeostatic and emotional control systems, especially within the limbic area.[5]

It is perhaps unnecessary by now to caution that the human brain, representing several hundred million years of compromises, is extraordinarily complex, and that mapping should not be taken too literally. That certain areas play a major part in sex, pleasure, or rage—and so on through a considerable list—cannot be much doubted; but we must always remember that each portion of the brain is part of an intricately woven and balanced system. The centers represent a concentrated mechanism involved in producing the complex changes and behaviors we call emotions rather than the source in any true sense. As in the case of the angry bull, the situation has to be identified as threatening before any emotions arise. Certainly the centers deep in the brain do not evaluate complex situations—that is work for the neocortex.

But if we look at a simplified cross section of the human brain, from front to back (Figure 6), we see the strategic location of the section called the thalamus. It was once the hind part of the front of the early brain's three lobes, and it acted as the head office insofar as the primitive brain had one. In the modern brain the thalamus serves as a busy, intricate crossroads, where major nerve pathways meet and mingle to some degree, and it contains important gray-matter switching centers that sharply influence where the flow of nerve-carried messages go, which get through, and which get blocked or shunted aside. The work of MacLean and other researchers has shown that the pathways through the thalamus and the surrounding limbic areas (limbic means bordering) are more complete and brain-unifying than was formerly believed.

Much evidence now indicates that the limbic area is, in general, the main switch in determining what sensory inputs will go to the neocortex, what decisions will be accepted from it, and which switches will be thrown locally. We can compare it to a switching tower in a freight yard that receives a flow of instructions from the main office

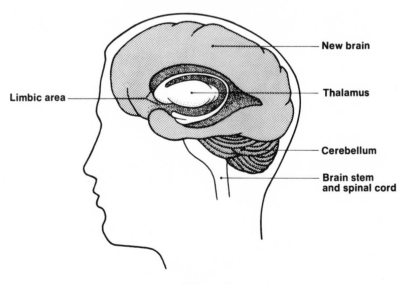

Figure 6

and follows them as a rule, but which may (if its crew decides the main office is wrong, or too slow, or not aware of what is happening) take over control and throw switches on local initiative. If, for example, the head switchman sees two trains heading for collision, he has no time to consult or argue—he quickly takes the action he thinks is right.

The thalamus and its associated centers step in and take charge when they sense grave threat, injury, or some sort of real or impending emergency that could affect survival. The implications of this, as we shall see in Part II of this book, are of the utmost importance in understanding learning and many other aspects of human behavior.

PART II

How the

Brain Functions:

An Introduction to

Proster Theory

CHAPTER 9

The Concept of Proster

I N its most elemental terms, Proster Theory sees human behavior as resting on a two-step cycle:
1. Choosing, from an existing repertoire, a program that best seems to fit the observed situation;
2. Putting the program into effect.

Typically, we decide, then act.

If in some instance an individual has only one course of action open (it is not easy to imagine such a case), then the decision would be automatic—but note that having no choice would mean not even between doing something and doing nothing. Automatic, "wired-in" responses are easy to find in lower level animals, and they may also exist in humans. We need not press the point, since obviously the vast bulk of our behavior does involve choice.

It is equally plain that if choice exists, action cannot take place until a choice has been made; and the choice must be made from *available* alternatives. I cannot escape an assailant by jumping into a car and driving off, unless (a) a car is there to use—the situation— and (b) I am able to drive a car—the program.

Suppose that a third party present sees that a car is there and could be used, but that for some reason I do not see it. So far as my behavior is concerned, no car is there, for what I decide to do is dependent on the situation as *I* perceive it; what other observers may see has nothing to do with me. In the same way, my ability to use a car depends only on whether or not I have the skill to operate it—what percentage of those present, or of the population, can operate a car has no bearing. Individual behavior is *individual*, but this appears to be the easiest fact to forget in dealing with or trying to understand human behavior.

At first blush the cycle of choose—act—choose—act may seem too simple to possibly be a base for complex and infinitely varied human behavior. If the first part of this book has served its purpose, however, it should be apparent that selecting from among a variety of alternative actions is precisely what makes a lot of gray matter necessary. To choose the action most appropriate to the situation implies evaluating or at least recognizing the situation and then matching an action to suit—perhaps selecting from several possibly appropriate choices. The evaluation of the situation and the selection of the action both have to be done in the light of the individual's past experience and his construct of the future. None of this can easily be shown to be unique to *human* brain functioning. Yet clearly man has not even a close rival in terms of the variety of situations he deals with, the subtlety of their differences, and the range and complexity of possible actions. As far as we know, no creature has a memory that rivals man's for storage of past experience, and even less for sense of future.

In the discussion that follows we will be building a model of brain operation. It need not be neurologically or electrochemically detailed or elaborate to serve effectively as the basis of a theory of learning and behavior. On the contrary, so long as it remains consistent with a more technical approach, a simplified model has distinct advantages, especially as we seek to apply it in practice. Our application is not brain surgery, nor even any kind of manipulation or exploitation of the brain's operation. Rather, we are seeking insight into how people behave and knowledge of how to reorder schooling so that it ceases to be an assault on normal brain functioning and instead becomes harmonious—releasing rather than inhibiting, helping rather than impeding, rewarding rather than frustrating.

As far as formal education is concerned, it can be sobering and useful to remind ourselves that, most remarkably, man somehow developed clothing, housing, tools, agriculture, pottery, superb art, writing, weapons and tactics, astronomy, and a good deal more long before the first grade was inscribed on the first report card or the first diploma handed over to give birth to the monster we now know as credentialism. Formal, institutionalized education is a recent and quite dubiously valuable development in man's history. When the human brain developed in response to needs, those needs did not include going to schools, passing examinations, or coping with bureaucracies.

Since the idea of proster is central to the model, let me explain the meaning of this invented term.

First, consider the idea of program. We live surrounded by a great variety of programs in mechanical form. For example, we insert bread in a toaster and push down the handle. This closes a switch to bring current to the heating element. In due course a thermostatic device responds to the heat, actuating a release—the toast pops up, and the current is switched off. This sequence is built into the toaster, and under normal conditions it will repeat hundreds or thousands of times.

A dishwasher has a more complicated program: once started, it rinses, drains, pumps out, goes through more cold water phases, then a series with hot water, and finally dries. Again, the program is built in, and will ordinarily repeat and repeat.

A phonograph record represents a long program that will deliver millions of consecutive bits of information to the stylus, resulting in a certain fixed sequence of sounds being produced by the equipment. Once the record is put on and started, we will get the same sequence of sounds again and again, modified only slightly by wear and conditions.

Program conveys the essential idea of a "frozen" sequence that does not provide for substantial variations. Even if we consider "branching" programs, in which alternative pathways are provided, the alternatives are fixed. (For example, in a certain computer program, normally number A will be bigger than number B, but it could happen that the subtraction called for cannot be made in some cases because B is larger than A. A branch may be provided, instructing the computer how to handle that situation—always, however, in the same way.)

But now consider a jukebox, that usually garish monster, which presents us with a choice of many programs. A large one can by ingenious mechanisms select any one of a hundred records, position it, and play that program. The programs it can choose from in response to instructions form a group with a good many features in common. All provide aural entertainment, by music, voice, or both together. All are in the jukebox presumably because they are suitable for use in the particular setting. Broadly, they serve the same purpose. Yet there may be good reason for a patron to select one rather than another—to hear one that is gay, or romantic, or suited to another mood, or to have music for dancing, and so on.

The jukebox represents a group of programs that are of a kind, all for the same broad purpose, yet offer alternatives because one may be more *appropriate* than others to a particular need at a particular moment. We can conveniently call this arrangement a "program structure"—or still more conveniently, compress that to "proster." As a new word, proster happily will not carry old associations or meanings.

Now observe my dog walking slowly along a path in the woods. Concentrate on the near rear leg. We can readily see a small program played over and over—the paw put forward, pushed back, picked up, put forward again. The other three legs have their programs, and the cerebellum, we know, is coordinating all four. We call this general program "walking." Now the animal begins to trot—the legs move faster and a little differently. In effect, he has put on a new record or shifted gears. I whistle and he runs to me, using quite a different leg action. If I now invite him for a walk, he will caper and gambol—still another shift of gears.

We can say that the dog has a proster for locomotion: a group of programs for the same general purpose from which he can select one to put into effect. This oversimplifies, of course, for we soon note that the dog has prosters at various levels. For example, if he is walking in the path and comes to a small log, he has to lift his front legs higher, and at just the right instant he lifts his back legs higher, too, over the obstacle he no longer can see. Clearly he has a program for getting over obstacles, a variation on his walking program. For the moment we can skip over these complexities while we first develop a basic model. This idea of program and proster is the key to understanding how the brain works, I suggest, and once we picture the human brain as a collection of a vast number of richly interconnected prosters, its functioning becomes enormously easier to comprehend.

For present purposes, we can represent a proster in diagrammatic, simplified terms (see Figure 7). As I forewarned, we are going to look at "thinking" as basically elaborate switching, with neurons being the brain's switches, sending an activating impulse message or not sending one; or, if having an inhibitory role, sending an in-

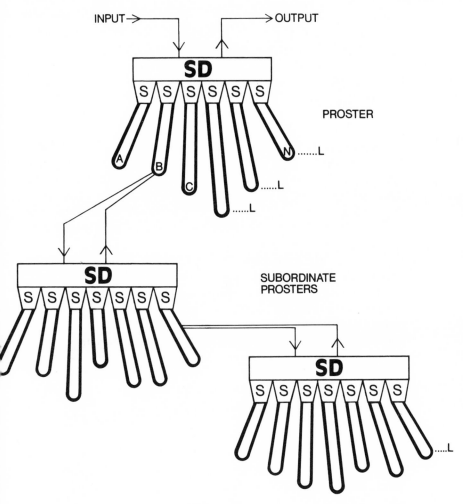

Figure 7

hibitory message or not sending one. (Sending is the switch's "on" position, not sending is "off." The same is true for the great numbers of inhibitory neurons, but here the message sent tends to keep some other neurons from firing.) Despite the complexity of the various kinds of neurons, this binary view appears consistent with present knowledge of the brain, at least for purposes of a general model.

An input signal enters the proster, going into a switching device (SD), within which one of several switches (S)—but only one at a time—can close, thus "playing" one of the attached programs, shown as loops (A, B, C, . . . N). Recall the jukebox, which can play any record in its collection, but only one at a time.

The programs within any one proster are always closely related, but the purposes of the millions of prosters in an adult brain cover a great range. By no means are all the "motor" type, as in this example of my dog's locomotion. Prosters can be seen as serving all the processes of thinking, all the brain's functions.

Programs A, B, C, . . . N may be said to be variations on a theme —or alternative ways of coping or alternative answers to a question. Any program in our initial proster may be linked with one or more subordinate prosters, as indicated for program B. In effect, this means that program B may be varied by cutting in any of the choices in the subordinate proster, which of course could have its own subordinate prosters—ad infinitum.

So far as this main concept is concerned, it does not matter whether the programs composing a proster are long or short, few or many, simple or complex through subordinates. What counts is visualizing the brain not merely as a mass of neurons but as neurons organized into this basic system of prosters, with millions upon millions of prosters having billions of interconnections. In Figure 7 (L) reminds us that all prosters are richly linked with others and most tightly linked with closely related prosters. This relationship, however, can be in many directions; for example, "tree" relates to leaves, green, wood, shade, forest, caterpillars, birds, specific kinds of trees or specific trees, tree as analogy as in family tree or coat tree, and many more.

The proster described is a model, not a localized, physical structure in the brain. It is put forward not as a neurological diagram but purely as a useful concept. What I have labeled "switching device" does express the effect produced by neurons in action. Elaborate gray matter is needed for cross-modal comparisons, such as decision making based on sight-sound, feel-smell, or multisensory inputs. Since different areas of the brain's cortex specialize in handling different sensory inputs, it follows that at least major prosters will *not* be localized, but instead are networks reaching into many regions of the cortex and, in at least some cases, into older gray matter. Prosters then may be thought of not only as the basic thinking apparatus, but also as the networks that, so to speak, tie the brain together.

When designing computers, electronic engineers seek to keep the circuitry as compact as possible, since reduced circuitry has an effect upon speed of operation. The electrochemical transmission along mammalian nerve fibers is enormously slower, the full range being about from one-half to 120 meters per second.[1] But though tiny "chips" of densely packed electronic circuitry not much larger than a punctuation mark can now be made, the most compact logic devices still don't begin to attain the density of neurons in the brain. The brain compares as an ox-cart to a space vehicle in speed, but compensates in density. And unlike the digital computer, which cannot handle many truly simultaneous inputs, the brain tolerates hundreds of thousands and can carry on a host of intricate simultaneous operations—a stupendous advantage. The kind of search that could be called "prostering" can go on quite rapidly, for practical purposes, because of this simultaneous feature. For analogy, suppose a diamond has fallen out of a ring at a party, and all thirty guests join in hunting for it, each taking a zone. The search proceeds far faster than if one person were doing all the searching, one zone at a time. The brain appears capable of carrying on a huge amount of simultaneous prostering.

Even at this stage, we can see the utility of the proster concept in illuminating human behavior. If we closely observe ourselves or others for a period, we can readily recognize this decide-execute cycle as being what we live by. Throughout the day, we switch on a program and "play" it.

I wake up in bed. I make a choice between rolling over for a little more sleep, lying awake awhile, or getting up. If I get up, I enter the bathroom and activate a complex group of ablution programs. I then must choose what I am going to wear. Having decided on a certain shirt, say, I execute a program involving many steps to open it up, put it on, and button it up. I go through similar choose-execute cycles with trousers and shoes. At breakfast, I choose what to eat and execute the programs for preparing or pouring or buttering, as well as eating. On some mornings I may fix myself either a fried or a boiled egg. Making such a decision early in the morning may not come easily, but the moment the choice has been made the program flows smoothly. In common language I would say if you queried me that "I do not have to think about it," meaning in proster terms that I do not have to "consciously" throw any switches. I merely let the program unwind.

During most of our waking hours we execute intricate programs "without giving thought." Observe a smoker. We see the decision to smoke being made, evidenced by the hand reaching into a pocket for a pack of cigarettes. One is extracted, tapped, put in the lips. A matchbook is located, opened, one match pulled out, struck, held to the cigarette, air is inhaled to effect a light, the match is shaken out and disposed of, the cigarette puffed on. Were we to analyze each detail of this sequence, the total would rise from the thirteen listed to perhaps fifty.

This program, we should note, is in actuality a proster, or collection of related programs, for the next time the smoker makes the same decision, the body may be in a different position, the matches in another pocket, the ashtray at another location. The series of motions must be modified accordingly. Since the adjustments are minor and the end result about the same, we can use the term program for convenience, so long as we remember that even what we may call simple actions are in reality so complex that we probably never in our lifetimes repeat one precisely a second time.

In the case of the smoker we may easily detect "loops." The hand reaches into a pocket, finds no pack, then recycles as an adjustment to try another pocket; or the cigarette does not catch at the first attempt to light and the lighting cycle is repeated. These loops are significant: they show that although the program is being carried out "without thought," feedback from the senses is causing switches to be thrown, but in prosters so many levels down that the choice is below "conscious" or "attention" level. As our first proster diagram indicated, any program within a proster can have its own subordinate proster, offering choices of just how that program will be executed; and in turn that subordinate proster can have, for each of *its* programs, more subordinate prosters, level after level.

For analogy, think of a general who orders an attack on a hill. In effect he has selected a program to be executed. His aide, a colonel, chooses how he will implement the order at his level. Further down the echelons, a major makes some smaller decisions, a captain still smaller ones for his command, a lieutenant for his men, a sergeant for his squad, and finally the individual soldier decides what ditch he will wriggle along and what rock he will take cover behind. The general soon loses sight of this process—many decisions are being made below his attention level. But his program is being carried out.

Our ability to give what we call attention is severely limited, as a variety of experiments have long since shown. We can focus on only a few items concurrently. Thus the hierarchy of prosters serves as an essentially simple, practical plan by which the brain can make a few big decisions at the attention or topmost level and have them executed by a sequence of subordinate prosters in which more and more detailed decisions are made at lower and lower proster levels.[2]

Let me stress the basic tenet of the theory: the brain is organized into prosters, the hierarchy of prosters represents the basic, pervasive mechanism by which the brain works. We perceive, recognize, evaluate, remember, think via level upon level of prosters.

Let us note that this system provides, as does the man-made computer, for branching or programmed alternatives for meeting common conditions. In the instance of the smoker reaching for cigarettes, the hand entering the pocket feels for the pack in the front of the pocket; if it is not found there, the program branches and fingers feel in the back portion; if nothing is found there another branching is cut in and the hand feels in another pocket. These are all pre-set alternatives, within prosters well below the attention level.

But suppose no cigarettes are found. In this case the program has been aborted, and an aborted program typically "sounds an alarm" that instantly brings the problem to attention level. This is a profoundly important mechanism that we shall examine in depth. For the moment consider what happens if you are walking along (executing a locomotion program) when suddenly your foot penetrates what seemed a solid surface, into a hidden hole. No matter what your attention may be on at that moment, the abortion of the walking program will take precedence.

Or suppose you reach for your wallet to pay for a purchase and find the pocket empty. You are likely to feel the effects of a surge of hormones responding to an emergency call—even if in an instant you recall that you deliberately left your wallet in a drawer and have cash in another pocket. In Proster Theory terms we would say that you had a scare not because you thought your wallet was lost or stolen, but because a familiar (and important) program was aborted.

Abortion of a program produces emotion because it is a *threat*; "Something is wrong!" How much emotion is felt, and of what kind, depends on the importance or implications of the program. Suppose I am taking a shower. Following my usual program, I step out and reach for the towel on the rack. But there is no towel there. Instantly I feel annoyance, quite possibly vented with an expletive. The abortion forces the problem to my full attention, driving out whatever I was consciously thinking about. I am now forced to rechoose a program at the attention level. I might call to someone to kindly bring a towel (program B), or go dripping wet to the closet to get one (program C), or raid another rack (program D), or otherwise find a program I can execute.

But now suppose I am not at home, but a first-time guest in a strange house, and my hosts are asleep. Lacking a program, I may find myself at least for a time confused, embarrassed, and immobile— I have no available program, I don't know what to do. The young, I suggest, often seem to older people either stupid or rude because they simply have far fewer established programs in their prosters. Lacking choices, they may appear silly, boorish, careless, or insensitive. Note too that in emergencies such as accidents, fires, explosions, and the like many bystanders often seem rooted to the spot. Either they have no preexisting program that can be executed, or the selection process has been for the moment inhibited. They do nothing; they may be described as frozen in their tracks. Unless they have a program to execute, there is nothing they *can* do but freeze. *No program, no activity*, in spite of tremendous "stimulus."

CHAPTER 10

Prosters in Action

AT THIS JUNCTURE, we can begin to define learning as the acquisition of prosters. And when we observe young children, the process of acquiring more and more programs, and more adequate, closely related collections of programs, or prosters, could hardly be more evident.

Here is a little girl in a highchair working hard at using a spoon. She turns it over, spilling the food, often misses her mouth on the first try—but with encouragement rapidly improves her control. If her mother tries to guide her hand to be helpful, the child will likely resist and grow angry. She much prefers to do it herself; if the mother insists on teaching, the child may well refuse to attempt to feed herself for several months. On the other hand, her obvious joy at succeeding leaves little doubt of how "motivated" she is to learn— her way. A few weeks later her spoon-feeding proster has developed so remarkably she can feed herself quite well even while her attention is elsewhere. The arm and wrist movements have smoothed out, control has become very accurate.

Here is a boy learning to use the index of a book. If he is allowed to learn his way, to make the decision to look up what is wanted in the index as well as to carry out the action, we will likely find him well-skilled in the use of many kinds of indexes a year later. If he sees a friend thumbing through page by page, he may grab the book away and use the index to speed the process.

The acquisition of prosters is not limited to any age. For example, observe an inexperienced young executive making his first major presentation to a meeting. Probably he is nervous, stumbles, jumps from point to point, fails to grasp the import of questions. But a few times later he functions smoothly, with poise, precision, and sensitivity to his audience. A fellow manager twice his age seated at a new and strange computer terminal takes ten minutes to painfully peck in a request for information. Later he can do the job in ten seconds and can if necessary instruct an assistant on how to get what he wants. An old man with a broken hip finds he has to learn how to get about his room in an entirely new way. Chances are he learns. So long as the brain continues to work, new prosters can be acquired.

We have no reason to believe that more than one basic process is needed for learning—for acquiring new prosters—or that it changes with age.

Becoming educated may be looked on not as acquiring knowledge, the conventional view, but as acquiring personally useful programs. As we have discussed, the *richness* of prosters develops along with the *number* of prosters and the *linkage* of prosters. The more variations on a theme a proster offers, and the more prosters there are, and the more densely they are interconnected, the more thinking resources we then have and the more choices are possible. Such a definition of educated, we may note immediately, carries enormously important implications. It provides a concept of learning that emphasizes variety of behavior—the polar opposite of the academic and training approach that implicitly seeks to narrow behavior to *the* approved, polite, or official form.

Growth is geometrical, in these three dimensions: richness, number, and linkage of prosters. This suggests why even slight differences in richness of prosters at birth can become major differences over a period of years, and why a deficit of input over a period can have a profound effect. Picture two similar children rolling snowballs. The one who begins with a slightly larger one will pick up snow faster, and the advantage will increase the larger the snowball becomes.

Even stated in such a preliminary fashion, this appears to be a simpler, more elegant explanation of a youngster's learning than the growth stages Piaget's work has popularized. It suggests why children with a reasonable starting fund of prosters and suitable input can so readily learn to read at age three and can read and compose at what is called "sixth-grade level" while in first grade—as Dr. O. K. Moore has brilliantly and conclusively demonstrated.[1] In recent years it has become vigorously evident that children can achieve important learning far earlier than traditionally they were thought capable of. Within education, where folklore serves so commonly as respectable wisdom, this has not of course served to dispel entirely notions about children's brains or eyes not being mature enough when they enter school. Should this nonsense somehow be knocked down, many teachers have a fall-back position: the child, they submit, should not be subjected to the pressure of learning. What they really mean, of course, is the pressure of teaching. To learn is precisely as natural and necessary as to breathe. To prevent or hinder a child from learning is the exact equivalent of interfering with his physical growth.

Assuming the inventory of prosters has been acquired, how is the right program selected from the many available?

Consider again the diagram of a single proster, with some additions (Figure 8). Note here the additional inputs to the switching device (SD), a, b, c, . . . n.

Recalling the discussion of homeostats and the term bias, referring to the setting of a homeostat (as we set the household thermostat that controls the heating plant), we can call these side inputs simply biases. These bring signals from elsewhere in the brain, which *in*

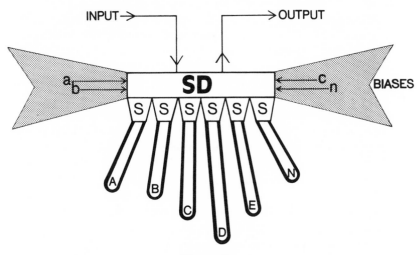

Figure 8

sum influence which of the selector switches (S) in the proster will be activated. Picture the parlor game in which the players sit around a table and try to blow a table tennis ball away from themselves and toward other players, who will be out if the ball goes off in front of them. The motion of the ball will reflect the sum of the forces acting upon it from different directions. A player who stops blowing can be said to be sending a minus signal to the ball, while one who is blowing is sending a plus signal. In much the same way, some of the bias inputs to a proster may be minus or inhibiting, while others may be plus or activating.

Or consider the general again, pondering whether to order the attack on the hill, one alternative open to him. Some of the information inputs he has received lead him to favor attack: he has the necessary forces, morale is high, air support is ready, the enemy has been under barrage and is believed to be tired and to have suffered casualties. On the other hand, they are well dug in, apparently have ample ammunition, and the hill offers a strong defensive position. Some considerations urge action, others inhibit. The sum will influence the decision.

Not only current information will affect the situation, however, but stored considerations will also: the life experiences that have made the general aggressive or cautious; the results of previous situations that he feels apply to this one; and his plans and ambition for his future.

The higher we go up in the proster hierarchy—the closer to the attention level—the greater the number of important bias inputs there may be. The function of the element in our model that we have called the switching device is to make a decision—that is, throw a switch—on the basis of the combined plus and minus biases received —and so select an appropriate program from the proster.

For the moment I am simplifying even the simplified model of brain operation. While my effort is to avoid neurological detail, the model is still consistent with current neurological knowledge. Neurons, the basic switches of the brain, take a number of forms, but typically a neuron (other than sensory) has many input branches feeding into its main portion, the cell body. These are called dendrites, a word deriving from the Greek for tree, for reasons Figure 9 makes obvious.

Dendrites connect with other neurons at a great many points— thousands and even tens of thousands in many cases. There are no actual joinings, but rather extremely narrow gaps across which a

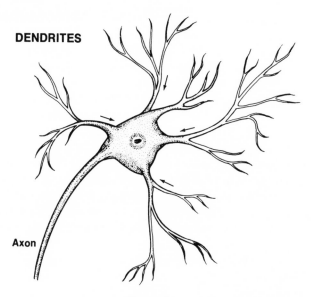

DENDRITES

Axon

Figure 9

transmitter may make a sort of chemical bridge for a very brief period, in effect closing a switch (which is, of course, essentially a gap) for a few millionths of a second. These gaps or switches are synapses. We can think of the dendrites as gathering binary information much as the roots of a tree gather nutrients.

The end of the axon, in most types of neurons, is also branched, often very elaborately. This is generally true of interneurons, those that connect to other neurons rather than to receptors of input from outside the brain or that carry orders to muscles or other organs of the body. These "afferent" (to-the-brain) and "efferent" (from-the-brain) neurons account for only a small percentage of all neurons. The great bulk of them are within-brain, devoted to processing information. (This fact throws light on the difficulties of the behaviorists, who at first assumed that an afferent stimulus was closely linked to efferent response. As it became apparent that simple links seldom existed, they introduced the now quaint term "mediation" to cover the gap—a gap now known to include most of the brain's apparatus!)

Neurons are typically all-or-none devices. Like a gun, they either fire or they don't. It now seems amply well established that firing or not firing depends very largely on the multiple, simultaneous inputs from a neuron's dendrites. Some encourage firing, some inhibit. (In electronic terms, a neuron may be considered a form of summing amplifier.)

While the analogy of a gun firing illustrates the all-or-none principle, a single discharge by a neuron has no effect. Only its continuing discharge—like that of a machine gun—will have any influence on other neurons. The rapidity or frequency of firing may have significance; and even more, changes in the rate of firing, which, by variations, can produce a pattern.

Numbering in the thousands of billions, synapses have a key role that still eludes precise definition, although much of the mechanism has been resolved in detail. Strong evidence has been accumulated that *graded*—in contrast to all-or-none—effects are produced within the neural network. This may sound contradictory, but for analogy think of a board of directors that has some progressive and some conservative members. Each has only one vote (all-or-none principle), but at various times two, three, four, or five of the progressives may vote together (graded effect). When more votes are cast for action than against it, it will be taken, and when more vote against than for, it will be inhibited.

This well-established basic brain structure suggests that the concept expressed by the proster diagram is substantially consistent with the actualities derived from neurology.

Consider once more the proster diagram (Figure 10).

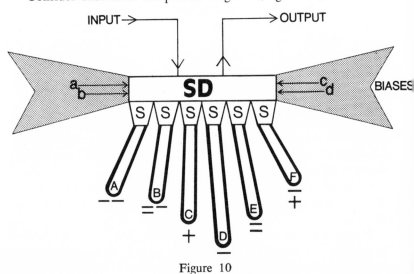

Figure 10

Let us say that in this instance bias (a) is strongly inhibiting the switches for programs (A) and (B), as indicated by double minus symbols (— —). Bias (b) is weakly inhibiting (—) switches for programs (B), (E), (F). Bias (c) is weakly inhibiting switches for programs (D) and (E). Bias (d) is weakly activating (+) for programs (C) and (F). Summing up, we see these totals:

(A)	. . .	— —
(B)	. . .	— — —
(C)	. . .	+
(D)	. . .	—
(E)	. . .	— —
(F)	. . .	0 (+ and — cancel out)

Under these circumstances, program (C) would be activated. If aborted, program (F) would be the next choice. (If all programs were inhibited by biases, the input to the proster would be refused and shunted out.)

To illustrate, only four bias inputs have been shown. In reality, there could be thousands, so the switching device would produce a far wider, extremely subtle range of values by which one or another program would be selected. For purposes of insight into behavior and fostering of learning, we do not really have to worry about the mechanism, once the concept of hierarchy of prosters is accepted, at least for use as a model.

I have used the word "appropriate" with reference to the choice of a program within a proster. Smith defines it succinctly:

> . . . The world is full of a restless energy: it is full, in Whitehead's phrase, of a constant and unending "stream of happenings." It is the animal's part to respond to these happenings in an appropriate manner: a manner, in short, which ensures the prolongation of its individual life so that its progeny may perpetuate that of the species.[2]

For man, this means ability to survive in a variety of settings, circumstances, and environments much greater than most other animals can tolerate. The uniquely manlike aspects of the brain must relate to unique origins and behaviors.

We can then define the human brain in one basic way as an instrument for perceiving, evaluating, and dealing with the situation in which an individual finds himself.

Let me make a distinction between *setting* and *situation* to avoid some serious confusion. I will use setting to mean a circumstance as it might be observed by various people, and reserve situation to mean only what is perceived by the individual under consideration. Situation is always unique; there is no way to be in any situation without bringing to it one's personal past and personal expectation of the future. Our physical receptors are personally unique: the colors and shapes I see are not identical to those you see, nor are tastes and smells and feel via my fingertips or inner ears. What is more, your prosters and mine differ in at least several million ways.

Most managers, educators, and others who must deal with many people tend, I think, to underestimate and underrespond to individual differences, because their work would be so much simpler if the differences *were* less important. Wish becomes father to thought: teachers give lip service to differences, but even the best often act to the contrary, forever trying to group students by "alikeness" rather than honoring the differences that have permitted the species to survive this long.[3]

Thirty children in a classroom are in the same setting, but each is in a different situation. Two children on a seesaw are in the same setting, but since each brings a different physique and experience, they may be in quite different situations—one gay and abandoned to pleasure, the other worried and hanging on for dear life, hoping to avoid the shame of being found afraid.

The word "percept" serves well to mean the strictly personal view of a situation. The appropriate choice of program then may be said to be that which best fits a percept. The dog in the woods selects his gait from his locomotion prosters in response to *his* percept. My response to the dilemma of the missing towel must be in the light of *my* percept—how someone else might see the setting has at that moment nothing to do with me.

The percept each one of us has normally seems so compellingly right that a sharply differing percept of another person in the same setting tends to seem incredible, or to offend us, or even to anger us—for the same reason that an aborted program rouses emotion. Two friends go to a play. One finds it absorbing and moving, the other finds it boring and trashy. The friendship suffers some strain. Husband and wife go to bed in the same room. One finds it stuffy and too hot, the other fresh and too cold, and each thinks the other peculiar, idiotic, or difficult for holding a differing view. The simpler the percept in question, the more clash develops.

The earlier years of formal education in particular are oriented precisely the opposite way. Constantly the child is taught that there is one right answer, with the strong implication that there is something wrong with the child whose percept leads to an unorthodox response. Shown a lump of coal, the child is supposed to say that coal is black. But the fresh eye of a youngster may see other colors present. (An adult may, too, by working at it very hard.) But black is the *right* answer, and the conventional school lives by right answers.

The percept arises from examination of the setting. As raw data, it must be evaluated before it can be acted upon, and the conclusions reached through evaluation will of course influence the selection of program in the light of experience, knowledge, and aims. And as we shall see, emotional factors in evaluation can greatly affect the way the percept is handled, and even the percept itself.

All three processes—perception, evaluation, and response by action —are aspects of the fundamental organization of the brain, the hierarchy of prosters. The brain is not a hodgepodge of mechanisms for handling "perception," "recognition," "associative thinking," "cognitive thinking," "affective thinking" (or "feeling"), "reinforcement," "memory," "recall," "problem solving," "concept formation," and so on through a ridiculous list—the equivalent of saying with a straight face that a phonograph has different mechanisms for providing us with the sound of vocalists, choruses, chamber music, jazz, soul, country and Western, poetry, speeches, and sound effects. These of course are outputs from varying records or inputs; the mechanism is the same for all.

Proster Theory suggests that the human brain has *one* basic mechanism, but it includes the basic mechanism at three stages of development: the reptilian brain, the less ancient limbic system (MacLean's old-mammalian brain), and the magnificent, dominant new brain, the neocortex.

The proster is common to all; it goes back to the very beginnings of brain. In a very practical sense, it is what we mean by brain, so far as function is concerned.

CHAPTER 11

Not Stimulus but Situation

Perhaps no word has done so much to make American psychology so unproductive a study as "stimulus."

The term, of course, is the very keystone of most systems of psychology that dominate the scene, and common to all. Yet it connotes two huge misconceptions that often guarantee that much that follows will be in error. Not surprisingly, we find on pressing the point that the various definitions of stimulus are exceedingly slippery. The term is used to mean energy or a force impinging on a receptor from outside the body or from within, or change in such energy, or some factor that alerts an organism in some way, or that acts as a sign or signal, or even a situation (setting or circumstance, by the usage I have suggested) that serves in such a fashion. The briefest examination reveals that such definitions aren't definitions at all, but circular reasoning. If I poke you and you pay attention, the poke was a stimulus. But if I poke you and you ignore it, the poke apparently was not a stimulus. This, we must agree, makes the usual notion of stimulus obstinately difficult.

To illustrate this oddity, Peter Nathan points out in *The Nervous System* that when a male trapdoor spider approaches a female there is no telling what may happen. She may respond to this stimulus by allowing him to live with her for some months, or tolerate him only briefly, or eat him on sight.[1] The problems of the male trapdoor spider with regard to stimulus would seem to be more worrisome than ours.

Day in, day out, in a hundred ways, we demonstrate that most stimuli, whether impingements or circumstances or signals, have value or meaning only as we give it them. We observe a magazine on a coffee table a dozen times and then pick it up to look at. Or we see a chocolate cake and refuse a piece, politely accept one next time, and eagerly serve ourself a large piece at still another. We hear a car backfire and pay no heed, but the next time we jump. We mislay eyeglasses or keys and find them lying where we must have seen them plainly, yet didn't see them.

The first false connotation of the word *stimulus* is that the organism is passive and will just sit there until a stimulus happens along. The second is that the brain responds to isolated factors, such as an electric shock, a light, or a bell. (Gestalt psychology, of course, has long resisted this general approach.) Although stimulus-response psychologists often tuck in disclaimers, the overwhelming impact of their writing and reporting, I submit, carries and continually builds these connotations. Who does not know of Pavlov's dogs, "conditioned" to salivate at the sound of a bell. But if a dog had been well fed and was on a routine walk, would the bell produce the effect? If his attention was on an approaching female in heat, would he then? Obviously, the bell was one factor in a situation offering dozens of potential stimuli. The dog *selected* certain of them. In fact, legend has it that at times the great Pavlov was heard to complain that the dogs tended to get conditioned to other factors, even to *him*.

In the shorthand of psychology, symbols of stimulus and response are often shown linked with an arrow, which of course points toward response. This in itself strongly suggests, each time it is used, the active nature of stimuli and the passive nature of organisms—precisely the reverse of reality. The brain is by far the most active part of the human body. Some 20 percent of glucose sugar-energy is consumed by the brain and 20 percent of the body's blood flow passes through it—amounts enormously disproportionate to the size of the organ.[2]

Further, the brain *has* to be active. Experiments have shown conclusively that if subjects are put in circumstances that sharply reduce the flow of input from the outside world (such as being shut in a soundproof cell or suspended in warm water) distress quickly becomes evident.[3] On a milder scale, all of us have experienced extreme boredom, with its concomitant restlessness, irritability, daydreams, and fantasies. Unless broken off soon, we feel a desperate need for input or activity. One of the problems on automobile assembly lines, for example, is the monotony that makes any kind of diversion welcome, even a violent quarrel or a wildcat strike. Bored women, isolated in the home, may turn to gambling, shoplifting, or extramarital activities—activities that significantly involve risk. In almost any conventional classroom, at almost any time, one can easily find students, not allowed to take risks intellectually, combatting boredom by taking the chance of being reprimanded or punished, sometimes persistently baiting the teacher. We must suspect that a great deal of youthful crime, violence, vandalism, incautious driving, and drug use arises out of boredom, however complex the causes.

Sports provide another large area of risk-taking and escape from routine—if the game can't be actually played, often intense fan identification offers a substitute. Almost any outdoor activity, especially hunting and water sports, introduces variety and risk. And travel, whether to the county fair, the isles of Greece, or the moon, automatically creates uncertainties and hazards.

The whole new science of ethology, which owes so much to the work of Konrad Lorenz, reflects a revolution against the old idea of stimulus. After long observing animals in natural activities, Lorenz had the temerity to scrap the long-established, "official" view of behavior as simply response to outside stimuli, and to see what he plainly saw—that, in Nathan's words,

> The brain leads the animal to seek from its environment the things that are necessary for its survival. . . . It is mainly the organ of motivation, the part of ourselves that makes us do everything we do.[4]

Desmond Morris, ethologist, zoologist, and at one time curator of mammals at the London Zoo, sees some vertebrates in particular, including wolf, raccoon, and primates, as "opportunists," who have evolved no specialized way of survival.

> In the wild, they never stop exploring and investigating. Anything and everything is examined in case it may add yet another string to the bow of survival. They cannot afford to relax for very long and evolution has made sure that they do not. They have evolved nervous systems that abhor inactivity, that keep them constantly on

the go. Of all species, it is man himself who is the supreme oppor-
tunist. Like the others, he is intensely exploratory. Like them, he
has a biologically built-in demand for a high stimulus input from
his environment.[5]

Some animals, including domesticated dogs and cats, have the
ability to turn down their brains after a spell of activity and doze
on the edge of consciousness, though easily alerted. Man, in vigorous
health, ordinarily does not. We sleep a limited number of hours, or
we are awake demanding input. Unlike many wild animals that
must spend a huge amount of their waking time either looking for
food or eating, ingesting nourishment only momentarily occupies our
full attention. (It was not always so—the invention of cooking, with
all its concomitant implications such as group meals, has been sadly
undercelebrated. Plucking berries off bushes or gnawing at fresh,
uncooked meat take hours and require attention. Fire applied to food
—which incidentally made agriculture feasible—gave our forebears
hours of daily extra time, and with it the need for new activity.)

This inner motivation, and the incessant demand for inputs (at
its peak in humans), plus the fact that we constantly execute long,
complex programs that are never precisely repeated, appear to under-
mine seriously the whole notion of conditioning and reinforcement.
These concepts rest almost entirely on laboratory experiments which
attempt to isolate certain inputs as stimuli. The isolation is usually
contrived and unrealistic.

Each of us lives in situations. Waking, we are in a succession of
situations, one flowing into the next—an unbroken stream of percepts constantly being modified. It is impossible *not* to be in a situation. Any stimulus is part of a situation and cannot be isolated in
any meaningful human sense.

Imagine a mouse exploring a kitchen in the night, and coming to
a trap baited with cheese. It investigates the cheese; the trap snaps;
the mouse is hit but not caught. Trembling, it recovers enough to
crawl to a hole. The trap was a very strong stimulus, apparently. But
was it? Our mouse, let us remember, is not a mechanic; it does not
understand traps, or why they are set out. It does not necessarily
attribute its near demise to this device of wood and wire. Perhaps
it has rarely gone into this corner of the kitchen—it went only because of the cheese. Now it may fear that corner, or the odor of that
cheese. Or perhaps there is a faint scent of gas in this area by the
stove, or possibly the floor was just polished all over and the mouse
will hereafter not tolerate gas nor venture on any floor that feels and

smells as this did. It may even be that the mouse went foraging this time at an unaccustomed hour, or while the television was on in the living room, or while a dog was barking outside. Which of these possible factors relate to the hazard it experienced it does not know.

Consider a young woman talking with an older one about a matter important to her career, which the older woman could help her with. Or imagine a real estate agent showing a house to a family. At the end of a half-hour the older woman seems uninterested, but the younger has no idea of what transpired to produce this result. The agent, too, can only make guesses as to why the family rejected his offering. Most human situations are exceedingly complex, and the flow of percepts makes them unstable. We all know the man who quarrels with his wife at breakfast and then snaps at the bus driver. We are not sure how much laboratory rats carry such grudges and bad temper and expend them on uninvolved victims, but we know humans do, frequently.

If I am enjoying a stroll in the woods nearby and suddenly find myself face to face at six feet with a skunk, I may react to this "stimulus." But what am I actually responding to? The sight of the animal has changed the situation as I perceive it. I thought I was safely enjoying nature, but a threat has appeared. Then I recognize the skunk as one often around and not likely to get excited at the sight of a person. My fear abates as I realize I need only avoid alarming it. I may even smile and try talking to it. Same skunk, different response. If the next day I see a descented skunk in a pet store, I realize at once that it must be safe to be on display. Same type of animal, different response. It is the situation (*my* percept) that matters.

I may well talk about this incident in the woods when I return home, because it was exceptional. If we review our behavior for twelve hours past, we quickly see that seldom does our percept change so dramatically, and rarely is the situation dominated by such factors as a mousetrap or a skunk. While unusual behavior may indeed be illuminating at times, the brain clearly must be suited to the conduct of usual behavior.

Nor can behavior be fractionated, as psychological experiments so often imply. We can exist in and deal with only whole situations. Educators, too, commonly forget this. They speak of a student "learning to read" or "concentrating on geometry" as though the student were not also in a school, in a classroom, surrounded by other persons, concerned about parental approval, and so on.

But the human brain is, to repeat, an instrument for perceiving, evaluating, and dealing with the whole situation in which its possessor momentarily exists. This situation constantly "flows" into modified or quite different situations. I may speak of going from the kitchen to the living room, but in terms of percepts I flow from one environment to the other. Sensory input changes a thousand times as I move. If I enter a dark bedroom and switch on the lights, the flow is not as apparent, because my brain knows what to expect. If it were a strange bedroom, I would have to look around it, and flow would be more apparent, so far as perceiving details of the room is concerned. But my basic percept, of being in a home, of entering a room, of having carpeting underfoot, of hearing street noise outside, of a myriad of such factors that tell me where I am and what is happening to my body, flows on without interruption. Only by rendering me unconscious can the flow be broken.

The human brain's handling of choice, or proster selection, is in response to continuous differential analysis of the individual's situation as perceived. The changes in the situation are what count, whether induced by external or internal events (I have suggested earlier that there is no clear boundary between those two classes). Not just one or a few but all the changes count.

When there is some dramatic or distinct element in the setting that looks like a stimulus in the common sense, it becomes easy to overlook this "all factors" aspect. Sitting in my car at an intersection, I see a red traffic light. It changes to green, and I go. It seems sensible to say the green light was a stimulus that made me proceed, but in truth this is not tenable at all. If a police officer were holding up his hand, I would not go, in spite of the green light. If the intersection were blocked or pedestrians were in the way, or another driver was threatening to beat the light, or I got something in my eye, or my engine stalled, or I was parked at the curb waiting to pick up my wife, I would not go. The red light going out and the green coming on represented only *one* change in my situation, *if* I saw it. (If I did not, it was not in my situation at all.)

We do not respond to stimuli, but only to changes in *total* situation, and then only as the changes are evaluated as calling for a new selection of program or proster. Think again of the proster diagram, of the dozens or hundreds or thousands of biasing inputs that affect the choice of program. To pay attention to one, and attribute the selection to it, is to lose sight of the whole system of activating and inhibiting balance. Stimulus is simply a troublesome term, arising not from life but from highly artificial, contrived experiments, and seemingly impossible to define in any but circular ideas. It seems the better part of wisdom to scrap it, and to suspect any system built on it.

The greatest damage from the use of this term may have occurred outside the field of psychology. Stimulus has become an everyday word, and with its use has grown the absurdly upside-down notion that our activity is in response to stimuli, and that the human brain acts simply as a receiver, passively waiting for something to be put into it. As we shall examine when considering "perception," the brain operates much like a radar, which sends out a powerful beam and analyzes what is reflected back. The brain aggressively explores the setting—even attacks is not too strong a word.

Implicit in this misconception lies a more subtle but equally wrongheaded aspect of stimulus—the notion of isolation *in time*. It is hard to find in psychological literature much reference to stimulus that does not assume it to be an almost instantaneous, one-time event, something parallel to a bullet entering a body, moving in one direction, once. Here again radar gives us a far more correct analogy: a rapid, back-and-forth, cyclic action by which questions are asked of the environment and answers brought back to be analyzed. This is a very different concept, which we shall now consider.

CHAPTER 12

Signals, Search, Perception

PSYCHOLOGIST and educator in general have rather rarely concerned themselves with the mechanics of perception. As we have noted, neither has had much stomach for going inside the head where the works are; and in any case it is pertinent to observe that in the last thirty years probably more has been learned about the deeper processes of perception than in all the period before. Looking inside is much more worthwhile than it used to be.

In daily life, we tend to assume that if we show people an object, they see it; that if we send some sound their way, they hear it; that if we offer some recorded message in any familiar form, they decode it. Yet daily we repeatedly trip over evidence that this often does not happen: we meet someone we know and fail to recognize him or her, or find that witnesses to some event grossly disagree, or discover a message has become absurdly misunderstood. Perception continually proves to be anything but automatic.

Only as we venture at least some distance into the technical processes by which the human brain handles perception can we begin to have insight into the seeming capriciousness of perception.

All perception input must pass along nerves. Although these vary in thickness and coating, nerves in general operate the same way.

Visualize fifty people standing in line two feet apart, handing bricks along one to the next so the bricks travel the entire length of the line in one direction. Each person provides energy, so the brick moves along at a uniform speed. There is an all-or-none effect: the brick can be passed or not passed—there is no other choice.

In similar fashion, nerves "hand along" impulses—in a manner quite different from the way an electric current flows along a wire or water flows through a pipe. Instead of flow, there can only be all-or-none impulses. A particular nerve fiber transmits each impulse at a fixed speed, so long as its diameter and coating remain uniform (factors that need not concern us at present). The term "nerve," we should note, commonly is used to mean a bundle of nerve fibers. The fiber is always part of a neuron, from several feet long in the instances of those that run to or from body extremities, to microscopically short in many other cases.

This transmitted-pulse arrangement gives us a binary system, made familiar by computer science. Conventionally, the sending of an impulse is represented by 1, and the opposite, or no signal, is indicated by 0.

A neuron cannot fire continuously. Since the impulse is electrochemical, the nerve cell has to "rest" briefly to recharge, so there is a maximum frequency (several hundred times a second) at which impulses can be repeated. Using our 1 and 0 symbols, this fastest rate would be 1010101010 . . .

A slower rate, with longer rests between impulses, could be represented 100100100100 . . .

Still slower would be 100010001000 . . .

A patterned firing, having a regular repetition, could be 1010010-10010100 . . . in which the "101"s are separated by "00." Or in 1010100001010100001010100000 . . . we easily see "10101" followed repeatedly by "0000." Obviously many and much more complicated patterns are possible. These merely indicate the principle.

We can also see that signal chains could take what we can call for convenience nonpatterned forms, such as 10100010010101001 . . . , which lack any quick repeats, and that any number of unique nonpatterned signals can be generated. As computers daily remind us, this binary system can handle an unlimited amount of information.

A computer is much restricted in its ability to receive truly simultaneous inputs. The human brain isn't. It can cope with millions of bits of information pouring in at any one instant. Some of these are filtered out at various levels before reaching higher centers of the brain (which we remember is three brains in a stack); others are simplified by being combined; those that still remain are distributed to many areas of the brain—which is another way of saying that the brain deals not with isolated input but always with very complex and rich input, with situation. It seems very probable that further reduction is accomplished by comparison.

As we know, if two singers or instruments produce almost the same pitch, we hear a slow beat where the two sets of waves reinforce each other. The principle applies to summing. Suppose the following inputs to be arriving simultaneously:

```
        100100100100100 . . .
        100010001000100 . . .
        101000101000101 . . .
        ─────────────────────
        301110202100301 . . .        (summing line)
          x    x x  xx x             (null line)
```

We see that the summing line produces a highly distinctive pattern, much as the letters of a word produce a pattern. This can then serve as a name or shorthand symbol for these three particular inputs arriving together—an identifying beat. (Note that the nulls, marked here by x, also form a pattern that could be recognizable.)

In turn, we could take two such summing lines and sum them, and continue this combining process so that thousands of input patterns in combination could be reduced to a few summing line (or null line) signatures. For rough analogy, we recognize a symphonic piece of music in which a hundred instruments are producing patterns by the combined, overall effect. More technically, the cone of the speaker that reproduces this music does so by a similar sum-and-null process. The single moving cone gives us the sound of many different instruments.

How do we recognize a face or a voice? Obviously we are getting very complex simultaneous input in either case, yet we can easily identify, not by "hard" detail, but by signature patterns that emerge from the mass of information received.[1]

These binary codes in their elaborate combinations are the only way information can get to the brain to be processed. We see by code, hear by code, feel by code, receive all sensory input by sequences of binary 1 or 0 signals. To know what the signals mean, to make sense of the huge input, we have to learn the codes, just as a telegrapher can make no sense out of a clattering instrument unless he knows the code being used. The telegrapher deals with one slow code sequence, the brain with millions flooding in simultaneously and far faster.

We see because light inputs reach the retina, where they are transduced into huge numbers of nerve impulses, which reach the sight center in the back of the brain, where the code patterns are interpreted (just how, neurologists are still far from knowing, although recent advances have solved a good part of the riddle).[2] Unless we know the coded signals, what the eye takes in lacks meaning. A person blind from birth who is enabled to see by an operation years later may need months to learn to tell a square from a circle by sight, even though he has no problem identifying each by feel. To recognize a square even then he may have to count the corners one by one, with some struggle!

We commonly see the same principle demonstrated in persons who have gradually lost their hearing. The older person who gets a hearing aid after years of increasing loss often is at first delighted, then disturbed. Apparently the decoding has to be refreshed as a skill, and patience is required, especially since the input cannot be fully a replication of natural hearing. Many find the task too trying, and the aid is abandoned. Those who persevere in time usually benefit. (The moral, of course, is to correct loss of input before it becomes severe.)

How are such coded inputs recognized?[3] For our present purposes we need not attempt to go too far into the technical aspects. Computers are quite capable of recognizing inputs in this way, even to the extent of being able to visually read numbers or letters, which are scanned and each reduced to a basic binary 1 or 0 code. More important to Proster Theory is the concept of "categorizing down."

This is familiar to us as the means by which mail reaches its destination. Consider one letter. The address is read by those handling the mail from bottom up. If from abroad, it is directed first to the right country, the United States, for example. Then it is routed to the right state and some distributing center, next to the post office for that zip code, then to the carrier who serves a neighborhood, who takes it to the right street and house number on that street, where it gets to the individual on the top line of the address. If it comes to a large corporation's office, it is categorized down to division, then to department, then to room, and finally to addressee. By this simple process of successively narrowing down the category, a letter can be directed so that any one of 200 million individuals can be selected, with the end result that the name on the envelope and the name of the person match up.

This organization, illustrated in Figure 11, is simply a version of the proster format we have already examined.

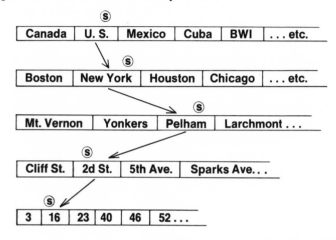

Figure 11

At each level in the hierarchy, the letter (input) is switched to one and only one of the many alternative programs; at the next level down the selection and switching is done again . . . at as many levels as necessary. If a recipient gets a great deal of mail, less of this selective switching is required. For example, a letter to "The President" can go directly to the White House. Nobody has to look for the city, or wonder what number on Pennsylvania Avenue it should be taken to.

This process of categorizing down can be called "search," for clearly the whole point is to find the match that is sought. The search permits some tolerance without doing violence to the scheme. For example, the letter in Figure 11 addressed to "Pellam" will still likely get to its addressee, and if the number has been set down as 15 instead of 16 it stands at least a good chance of delivery. If the error goes beyond the tolerance, an abortion of program occurs. Or if mail is addressed to a street or house number or person that doesn't exist, delivery of course cannot be made. No *match* is possible.

This search process, via categorizing down, via a hierarchy of prosters, is the *basic* way we recognize coded sensory inputs. It is what we mean when we say perception. If there is a match, perception ocurs; if no match can be found by the search, there is no perception—at least, not from this particular input.

We are so used to thinking that if we look at something we see it, that at first this concept may seem baffling. Yet daily experiences constantly illustrate the principle. Suppose three people are standing around a car: an auto mechanic, the woman owner, and the Brazilian tribesman who has never seen a car before. They lift the hood and all look into the engine compartment. The mechanic at a glance sees a great deal and observes that the distributor cap is loose; the woman sees the motor, air intake, fan and belts, and not much else; the Indian sees nothing but a snarl of vague shapes. For all practical purposes *what we "see" is only what we can recognize.*[4] As the once blind but now sighted individuals prove, even the simplest forms and shapes have to match up with "samples" in the brain, acquired through learning (a few may be at least partially present at birth) or they can't be seen in any meaningful sense. The same must be true for all other sensory inputs.

Jean Piaget's studies have called attention to the fact that young children up to about seven years of age cannot as a rule even copy moderately complex geometric or other shapes with much success.[5] Apparently some mental image must preexist that enables the material to be copied to be seen before the motor copy can be effected. As many parents of young children are aware, children of three or four can often copy circles with ease, but may not manage a decent square until around five, and a rotated square, or diamond, may take two years more to accomplish. Motor difficulties can hardly explain this— the circle is probably most complex—but the square requires the concept of straight lines meeting in a pattern and the diamond that of rotating a figure. The child is born with a schema for "face" that is close to a circle—children draw faces as circles for many years. An adult without art or some similar visual training (which provides a repertoire) can have great difficulty copying a free, abstract design that cannot readily be analyzed into familiar component forms.

In the analogy of mail delivery—and the game of Twenty Questions played expertly provides a similar one—the categorizing down proceeds linearly, along a single track. We must note that the brain categorizes down simultaneously along a great many tracks, usually involving more than one modality—which is simply to say that our various senses help one another interpret the environment.

Suppose you are seated before a large heap of strung beads. Some of the strings are short, others of differing lengths. The beads are of various diameters; some round, oval, tubular, or multisided, with others faceted; some smooth, others rough, some dull and others shiny; and they are of a dozen colors. Some strings are fairly homogeneous, others show pattern repetitions, still others evidence a random mix. Now one strand is put before you, and you are asked to find a matching strand in the heap.

At a glance you will see that there are many ways to approach finding a match. Your sample string is medium length, so you can categorize out all short and long ones. It has all smooth beads, so any that contain rough ones are out. It includes several shapes, so strings containing only one or two shapes are out. The predominant color is blue, so those not showing the same dominance can be excluded. Now suppose that some of the beads have quite a distinctive odor, and still others are hollow, and rattle. This would extend the parallel categories into two other modes, smell and hearing.

With some experience, you could probably do some parallel sorting. You would not have to sort out all the medium lengths, and then of these all the smooth ones, and then of these all the mainly blue ones—instead, you could choose or reject on two or more of the criteria at once. This would be (almost) simultaneous categorizing. The brain handles an enormous amount of simultaneous categorizing and categorizing down so long as attention is not required and lower-level proster hierarchies are doing the job. Tens of thousands, hundreds of thousands of such processes can go forward literally simultaneously within the brain's billions of neurons and trillions of proster connections, within one mode or much more, usually within several modes.

For this reason, perception normally appears to occur with no time lag; but many experiments demonstrate that a perceptible lag does occur. We have to get a good look at an unexpected object to know what it is. If a picture is flashed on a screen for only a small fraction of a second, we may be able to say that we saw a picture but not what the subject matter was. Only because the brain can process great amounts of input simultaneously can we perceive as fast as we do, and even then, as we shall shortly discuss, the brain makes use of a major shortcut.

The persistent popularity of psychologies built on the notion of active stimuli rather than active, aggressive brains also contributed to the assumption that stimuli were not only "outside in" in direction, but also one-stroke, one-way activators. But today the concept of feedback is well established. We perceive in a *continuous* process, as we flow from situation to situation. Our brain's interest is in changes in the situation. And via feedback and a constant questioning of the environment, humans in good health vigorously probe for the information they need to live by.[6]

How do we steer a car down a road? We turn the steering wheel what seems the approximate amount required—the tyro's guess may be far off the mark, the experienced good driver's estimate very close —and then see what happens. If the car is veering to one side, a correction is made; the effect of this is noted and further correction made. The good driver makes many corrections, so continuously and smoothly, with little if any overcorrection, that the back-and-forth procedure of asking "How am I doing?" and getting the answer does not become apparent. Yet if one watches the hands on the wheel, the frequent tiny corrections can be readily noted.

If I go up a flight of stairs, I activate a much-used locomotion proster that enables me to lift each foot in turn to just about the right height to come down accurately on the next step above, but it is the feedback from the increasing pressure on the sole of that foot that permits me confidently to shift my weight to it. Reach up with thumb and forefinger to grasp the lobe of your ear firmly. Feedback from receptors, thousands of them, in arm and hand, give you knowledge of where your thumb is in relation to your ear; and as you grasp, the pressures on ear and fingertips tell how hard the muscles are squeezing. At every instant in these actions information is flowing both to and from the brain, and each flow is influencing the other.

The same is true in "outside" perception. Our receptors are not passive mechanisms, slaves to outside inputs. To quote Pribram, one of the relatively few investigators to wed psychology and neurology:

> A great deal of work has been done to show that the activity of all receptors, or at least the input channels from them, is directly controlled by the central nervous system. These "gates" allow the organism to be sensitive only to certain excitations—the gates in turn are self-adapting mechanisms, i.e., they are subject to gradual alteration by the very inputs they control.[7]

Perhaps the simplest way to illustrate this from daily activity is to observe that what we possibly can see is continually sharply limited by which way our head is oriented and which way our eyes are turned, matters decided by us rather than by our environment. We continually select what we will look at, and the procedure is far more complex than simply turning to look. To illustrate, suppose something barely within our vision moves. Many receptor cells in the retina (technically a part of the brain) are linked so that groups will fire in a certain sequence if a moving object causes a change in the light falling on them. They not only detect movement, but the particular sequence signals the direction of movement. Now an old part of the brain computes how head and eyes (and if necessary, neck and body) must be turned to focus the moving image on the fovea, the sharp vision portion of the retina—a neat bit of rapid calculating. At the same time, feedback systems or "servomechanisms" adjust the iris to admit the desirable amount of light. Actual seeing now begins, as patterns from many groups of receptors in the retinas are sent to new portions of the brain in the extreme back of the head for analysis and synthesis, based on comparison with stored patterns. In infinitely more subtle ways, the nervous system controlling our sight will *inhibit* certain groups of receptors (or the signals from them) in order to sharpen perception of what is preliminarily "suspected" of being an edge. The light that falls on the retina is not what we see, but only the raw input from which the brain, instant by instant, will select information that seems useful in terms of the current situation and past experience.

Proster Theory suggests one cannot quickly shed old notions of perception in the course of reading a few pages. Some readers may feel that it is bad enough to have computers as prevalent as they are, without having millions of binary codes in our heads being the means of viewing a sunset or listening to Bach. To understand better how humans behave and how we learn, however, we have no choice but to deal with the brain as, to the best of present knowledge, it actually operates. To summarize the essentials:

1. The nervous system can internally transmit sensory inputs only in the form of binary code.
2. The codes can be simplified by summing.
3. To perceive, the codes must be recognized.
4. Recognition by matching is obtained by categorizing down through many levels of prosters.
5. Categorizing down can proceed simultaneously along many paths and in different modalities.
6. Reception of information is not a one-way, outside-in process, but a back-and-forth, radarlike process.

7. Receptors are not "automatic," but either they or input channels from them are constantly controlled by the brain or spinal cord.
8. Feedback, a continuing process, guides us in relating to our environment.

It may be worth noting that this scheme of perception gives a ready explanation of what has long been a baffling problem in many psychologies—and a strong hint that they were far off the mark. How can we recognize a cow, a bicycle, or a teaspoon, when we see these at different distances, so that the images projected on the retina must be many different sizes? How are we able to estimate size, when a large tree or airplane a long way off appears smaller on the retina than a small tree or airplane that is nearer? And how can we identify a spoon when it forms a differently shaped image on the retina according to whether we view it broadside, or head on, or end on, or at an angle, or from above? The Proster Theory answer is that we do not recognize what we are seeing (to use that modality for example) any one way, but because the categorizing down goes on simultaneously through many hierarchies. We identify cow or bicycle or spoon because we are getting inputs in code form on shape, color, texture, motion, and other attributes. The setting helps us enormously because it usually indicates relative size and gives strong hints as to what we may expect to find. With experience, we enrich the prosters by which we recognize a spoon or other object at many angles. But since recognition goes by codes, by patterns of impulses, tolerance is built into the system. We do not need an exact match to perceive— an approximation will do, just as a tune hummed with a number of errors or off-pitch notes may still be quite identifiable. The tolerance increases as simultaneous prostering goes forward; six approximate matches make correct identification much more probable than two approximate matches, sixty much more probable than six.

Brain researcher Mary A. B. Brazier, observing that many brain investigators have suspected the probabilistic nature of the brain's workings, comments:

> The margin of safety that the brain has for acting appropriately on a probabilistic basis would be much greater than that which would be imposed by a deterministic arithmetically precise operation. Chaos would result from the least slip-up of the latter, whereas only a major divergence from the mean would disturb a system working on a probabilistic basis. The rigidity of arithmetic is not for the brain. . . .[8]

For a century many psychologists have attempted to investigate the brain (from the outside) by simplifying, by creating experimental settings in which, hopefully, one variable at a time can be observed. (Since this is hard to do with humans, animals were much preferred as subjects.) This is something like removing one note from a symphonic piece and trying to learn from it in isolation how it functions. The brain, especially the human brain, operates as a fantastically complicated device. It is by evolution multiphased, comparative, evaluative, and only by accepting that fact as an investigative premise can we hope to learn how it works. We cannot simplify perception; it occurs *because* many prostering procedures are going on simultaneously amid the brain's billions of neurons.

The organization and stored content of those brain cells are unique in each individual, and the differences from person to person prove enormous. A trained copy editor will quickly spot a typographical error that most people might miss. But put him on a desert trail with an experienced tracker, and the tracker will read messages in the sand and rock that the copy editor cannot see even after they are pointed out to him. Almost all perception is *learned*.

CHAPTER 13

From Clues Compared,
Recognition

T HE BRAIN, being aggressive, constantly investigates the environment. We have to keep reminding ourselves of its intricacy and capacity, especially when we are indulging in simplifications in the effort to understand it. In the retina of one eye, for example, the rod and cone receptors number about 130 million. Other receptors by the tens of millions provide the inputs we know as smell, hearing, touch, heat or cold, pain, and motion sensations. Millions more tell the brain where the various parts of the body are, what stresses the muscles are under, and how they are moving.[1] It is probably fair to say that more information is being handled by the central nervous system of one's body at any given moment than, in terms of "bits," is being transmitted by the entire United States telephone system.[2]

Input must be filtered. Much of this process is attributed to the reticular formation, deep in the hindbrain and into the midbrain, and accordingly very old in evolutionary terms. This tremendously complex and diffuse network (reticular means netlike), being old, has primary concern with arousal, autonomous, and motor matters, but it can also pass signals through to higher centers in the midbrain limbic areas and to the new brain. What is allowed to pass, and where it is directed, must be assumed to take the form of a reciprocal arrangement, probably much like that of any office mailroom that sorts and distributes mail according to a standard operating procedure, but which could at any time be instructed to divert certain kinds of mail to, say, the auditors, or to delay certain packages pending return of an executive, or to rush any mail received from a certain source. In exceptional cases or circumstances, the mailroom might ask for instructions, or receive orders to consult or report progress.

Here again we can see that the proster kind of switching device can serve the purpose. Circumstances of the moment change the organism's needs, and the bias inputs to the prosters shift accordingly, routing the inputs being handled in different ways at different times. For example, normally the slightest burn on any part of our skin will be transmitted immediately to our attention, since it calls for action. But if a father rushes into a flaming house to rescue his children, he may not become aware of burns until he is out of the house and recovering from his intense effort. The burn information was biased out under emergency circumstances. Biasing out can be extremely subtle as well. Our brains are most limited in ability to "give conscious attention." In contrast to the staggering volume of information and procedures the brain can handle simultaneously, attention seems capable of encompassing perhaps half a dozen items at most, and quite possibly even this is managed by rapid sequencing rather than truly simultaneous handling, as is typically done by a digital computer handling many tasks at once.

In selecting what information will be processed how far, the entire system—quite sensibly, we might observe—ignores a vast amount of input that is not useful or productive. As the aggressive brain attacks the environment, the entire perceptual apparatus concentrates on what is recognizable, or almost recognizable, via binary codes, to existing prosters, and usually brushes aside the rest as meaningless to *this* brain. If for example we hear two voices in the next room speaking a language utterly unintelligible to us, we may have some interest in the voices themselves and emotional overtones, but we find it virtually impossible to keep attention on the language. Should we attend a lecture on an unfamiliar topic so esoteric that we can't make a grain of sense out of what is being said, we experience the same effect. In conventional schools, students who have "turned off" unproductive talk this way are usually readily visible. Teachers may call them inattentive or unmotivated, not realizing that they have no choice: the brain demands that they find more productive input, even if only daydreaming or watching clouds through the window.

In many circumstances unproductive input that cannot quickly be grossly identified (as we know that a foreign language at least is a language) produces alarm, fear, or the urge to escape. For example, the experienced driver of a car that suffers a flat tire will instantly identify the sound and know what has happened. But the new driver may perceive no more than noise not normally a part of the driving situation, and may well feel actual terror.

Even with filtering and selection, the input to the brain remains huge. We have many indications that the problem is met by extensive use of "clueing."

In daily life we use the device of clueing incessantly by giving things names. One doesn't have to say, "the city of eight million people located where the Hudson River flows into the Atlantic," when just "New York" will serve. "Henry Higgins" will clue a particular person, for most purposes. But clues inherently provide only tentative identification: New York could mean the state. Several people might have the name Henry Higgins.

Because the brain is an extraordinary comparative, differential instrument, it can use very slim clues with high accuracy. Say a large animal is approaching, brownish in color, that clomps as it trots and has a certain scent. A set of such fragmentary clues add up to "horse," even though in another instance the animal might be a good deal smaller, produce a neigh instead of clomp, and be pure white. We recognize a person we know in spite of great differences in dress, grooming, position, setting, or activity, even at times when we get only a distant glimpse, or when we see a poor quality black-and-white photograph. (This common experience makes the usual meaning of stimulus very baffling indeed.) Obviously no simple one-to-one recognition explains this. The comparative-differential structure of the brain does readily explain it: the brain is organized, via prosters, to compare the results of simultaneous input processing and to deal with differences or change.

Figure 12 suggests in simplest terms how clues can be cross-checked. Assume a St. Bernard dog is the object being recognized, and along one proster hierarchy it has already been categorized down to animal. Along other proster channels, *size, sound made,* and *coloring* have each been partially categorized down, not to a single match but to a few possibilities—not by detailed examination of the dog but by quick, rough, evident clues.

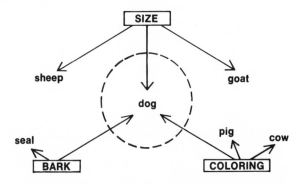

Figure 12

The rough clue *size* could fit sheep, dog, or goat; the bark could be a clue for seal or dog; the coloring suggests pig, cow, or dog. But only "dog" fits all three clues. Since this dog is unusually large, confirmation may be sought for the tentative finding of "dog." The viewer's eyes may be instructed to examine the shape of head or feet, location of ears and eyes, or the hand may feel the fur, or the animal's mode of movement and behavior may be prostered down and matched, still by relatively crude clues. The greater the number and variety of clues, the more certainly do clues serve to identify. What we might call the main track clues—the most obvious and familiar—will likely be categorized down faster and comparatively analyzed before a second, third, or fourth round of perception brings in confirming clues more rare or subtle.

Perception is then a gradual, qualitative, continued process, rather than instantaneous or all-or-none. In simplest language, the longer we observe the more we see, the longer we listen the more we hear— if additional prosters can be categorized down to utilize additional clues or input, if more binary codes can be matched in prosters. Looking at or listening to something totally unintelligible for a longer time will do no good if no fresh clues are received. Ordinarily, the process of utilizing the first, more obvious clues, then obtaining second or third or more rounds of confirming clues, all takes a mere fraction of a second.

Bird watching, that often denigrated hobby, has a chastening effect on those who think perception is a simple process. The beginner may be shocked to discover that he cannot even find the bird more experienced observers are exclaiming over, unless it flies away—in which case the opportunity to study it usually flies off with it. Once the bird is located, even with binoculars, it can be exceedingly difficult for the watcher who lacks sharp mental images of the various birds in the region (which is to say well-stocked prosters) to observe clues, in the brief glimpses possible as the bird moves on a branch or flies close by. What was the shape of the bill? Was there a tuft on the head? How many wing bars? What shape and color was the tail in flight? The neophyte can only say, "I didn't notice." Meaningful perception depends on recognition, recognition on preexisting prosters.

Consider a group of experienced bird watchers as they spot a bird on a high branch. "Yellow breast," reports one. This clue categorizes down significantly, eliminating scores of varieties that do not have yellow breasts. "Right size for a warbler," suggests a second, categorizing down on another hierarchy. "Could it be a female tanager?" asks a third viewer. Clues are now sought along this line. "No, it's dark on top, and greenish." Another adds, "The tail seems long for a warbler." "My hunch is a yellow-breasted chat," submits the group's expert. "Has it a dark sharp bill and a white line to the eye?" New clues are looked for, and found as the bird turns around. "Yes, I can see the head—sharp bill, white line." The bird is now fairly well identified. Note the process: the watchers gathered clues, went back for more, kept categorizing down, finally found enough clues to justify a comparative, cumulative identification. The whole procedure is analogous to that the brain employs.

Clueing is so valuable a shortcut that we can assume the brain uses it as standard operating procedure—a conclusion that the many well-known experiments on closure or completion strongly support. If we can read fast, it is by clueing—not by examining each letter or even each word. If we quickly see the nature of an arithmetic or geometric problem, or at once grasp the point of a joke, it is by clueing.

Since the ability to clue effectively depends on what is already stocked in recognition prosters, the ability of individuals within a group to clue from specific input may well vary over virtually a 0 to 100 range on this ground alone. (As we shall see, there are emotional factors, too.) These differences obviously are of enormous consequence in any kind of training or teaching; yet we may suspect that few teachers give much thought to perception at all, and that most assume that if they hold up an object, or play a tune on the piano, then all thirty students before them will see or hear the same thing. They don't. Each has his or her own, personal perception—no two alike. In addition, each likely is clueing from the teacher's tone, manner, movements, posture—from a host of nonverbal and situational inputs, most of which the teacher is not even aware of providing. These unintended clues may lead a student to proffer the answer wanted, totally without use of the information the teacher is trying to present!

Our human brain is not a simple unit mechanism but rather a stack of three brains; and as we examine the processes of perception further, we have to consider the role and influence of the older portions. Before we leave this basic discussion of clueing, however, let us note that Proster Theory suggests that:

1. The great bulk of ordinary, daily, operating perception is via the superficial, multicomparative shortcut of clueing.

2. Unless existing prosters contain at least rough matches for potential clues, in the form of binary code patterns, the individual cannot receive the clue. The mere fact that the energy represented—for instance, the light waves or sound waves—impinges on his receptors does not mean that any clueing or recognition resulted.

3. Since each individual has his own personal, unique inventory of prosters at any given time, no two individuals in a common setting will clue and perceive in the same way or to the same degree, and the range of clueing effectiveness can be from 0 to 100 percent.

4. Clueing is a back-and-forth procedure: clues are received and categorized down; more clues are sought to resolve uncertainties; more clues are received and categorized down—until by comparison and differential analysis tentative perception is achieved. The longer the back-and-forth process continues productively, the more reliable the perception becomes.

CHAPTER 14

Surviving as a Human Being

Proster Theory[1] holds that the proster, a multiple switching device, biased by the summing of side inputs and arranged in long hierarchies, can schematically represent the basic organization of the brain. Thus far we have examined the concept of motor programs arranged in prosters, the choice of an "appropriate" program from those in the inventory being effected by the biasing which results from comparative-differential analysis of the situation as perceived; and the use of prosters in the process of perception by which this comparative-differential analysis is made. Later we shall deal with memory, and it will already be obvious to the perceptive reader that the process of storing information in memory and recalling it when needed can be viewed as another application of this proster organization. It may also be evident, at least in a general way, that what we call "creative thinking" and "problem solving" can also be explained by proster switching.

We are all terribly handicapped in trying to understand how our brains work by the damage that has been done by conventional experimental psychologies. For a century, thousands of busy and often influential laborers in the tangled jungles of mind have aimed, manipulated, schemed, and at times fought with claw and insult to fractionate human behavior for study purposes. As we have noted, most have preferred to work with much simpler-brained animals. Only recently have the ethologists broadened their field and begun to have some compensating influence toward studying natural and complete, as well as comparative, behaviors.

If we go to the zoo to study various animals, we may learn—and be able to prove in fully documented papers—that some spend most of their waking hours pacing back and forth rhythmically at the front of their cages, and do not engage in productive copulation with the opposite sex even when encouraged. The second observation, if not the first, should lead to some suspicion that studying *caged* animals may not lead to reliable conclusions about the nature of these creatures. Trying to explain how a species survives for many generations without breeding young is sticky, even for a fully credentialed behaviorist. Yet the behaviorists, wholly unabashed and even militant, fill volumes with observations of caged creatures, some of them human, and try to sell us the results as valid and illuminating. Educators, particularly in the lower schools, engage in the same practice. When I asked one experienced teacher whether in her twenty years of school work she had ever dealt with children outside of the cages called classrooms, she appeared to consider the question offensive and did not reply. In fact, she has not spoken to me since.

With rare exceptions, teachers in our conventional schools do not often see their students' behavior as responsive to the prison they are in, the school; the cell they are in, the classroom; and the behavior of the wardens, the teachers. Rather they commonly say, "Arthur has a very bad temper," without adding, "in my room." Or "Julia shows little interest in her work," instead of, "in the work I assign her." Or "Edward has a surly, antagonistic attitude," but not the more accurate, "attitude toward *me*, in this class he is forced to attend." To some degree this no doubt occurs because the teachers mean well and believe they are trying to help, and that the child must accept the cage he has been thrust into, if he or she is to get along respectably in society.

But despite the efforts in this book to simplify brain structure and operation, we must keep reiterating that the brain is staggeringly complex, and that being a comparative-differential device, it deals with complex situations naturally and with contrived, would-be simple situations unnaturally. I do not mean to suggest that nothing can be learned from structured experiments or from confinement settings;

I do mean to stress that any findings from such sources must be regarded with suspicion, and verified by observation in natural situations.

To use comparative analysis, the brain must have two or more elements in which to find matches, and to apply differential analysis, two or more in which to find differences. As inputs to the brain number millions of bits per second, these processes minimally involve thousands of factors, processed simultaneously along hundreds or thousands of proster hierarchies. This is not an operation we can simplify by putting a pigeon in a Skinner box.[2] For a partial analogy, we can picture a group of racehorses thundering around the last turn and into the stretch. Watching them, we can see which is leading, which is threatening to take the lead, which is coming up on the outside, which are falling back under the pace. This is clearly a comparative-differential view—where the horses are means nothing, only their position in relation to one another, and the changes in that relationship which are becoming apparent. Contrast to this a single horse training at dawn, racing against the clock. Only remotely can we learn anything about the first kind of event by examining the second. (Even if the single horse's time indicates whether he might win or lose, we cannot be sure that in a race conditions might not influence him either to run slower, through being blocked, or faster, by being inspired by competition—or that any of the other horses might not do better if pushed.)

We also need to remind ourselves that we have not one well-designed brain, but an unplanned, improvised (though time-tested) arrangement that results in three brains of different evolutionary ages occupying one skull. Like a family in one house, they live together but don't always get along too well. In most psychologies one finds scarcely a mention of this fundamental fact of origin, and almost no concern for the interplay that results. We must deal with the brain not only as a device evolved to cope with complexities, but as one in which constant contention goes on as new situations are perceived.

As a broad rule, the older the part of the brain, the more it is concerned with maintaining the body's routine functions and homeostats, and the simpler its response to environmental input. In proster terms, it has relatively very few prosters, and these hold very few programs. We can throw some light on our reptilian brain if we consider how little choice of motion a snake or turtle has. We can also be sure, from the amount of brain equipment it has, that it gathers, by our standards, only a crude, limited picture of the environment—MacLean's imagery suggests a murky, low-resolution television screen reporting the outside world as perceived. It has relatively few recognition prosters, so that much of what it sees or hears can be categorized down only to various vague shapes or sounds. Those sensory inputs most important to survival, we can confidently assume, are the best perceived—but most important here means to the species, not the individual.

This brain, limited as it may appear, serves the creature not only in respect to breeding and obtaining food but in a long list of activities such as hunting and homing, finding shelter, and perhaps in relations with others of its kind. But this brain, in MacLean's words, is "filled with ancestral lore and ancestral memories and is faithful to doing what its ancestors say, but it is not a very good brain for facing up to new situations."[3]

Surrounding this brain in humans (as in all mammals) is the much more sophisticated and subtle old mammalian brain, or limbic cortex. As much fairly recent work on the brain has often dramatically shown, the structures here are intricately linked to what we generally call "emotional" feelings and behaviors. Since the linkage between the various portions of the entire brain is complex and ties the whole together, we cannot think of any element as separate in function; but for our present purposes we can consider the reptilian brain to be the one concerned with the oldest, most elemental emotions of utter rage (fight), utter fear (flee), and basic sexual urges, built-in for species preservation. The old mammalian brain greatly elaborates what we call emotions, and the huge new outermost brain again elaborates them to a great range of subtle feelings that to a degree can be verbalized. The cerebral cortex (especially its front portion) appears quite plainly to exercise a control over the behavior that emotions might otherwise cause. The interplay between our new brain and the old mammalian region is of the utmost importance to Proster Theory. The relation to the reptilian brain is of consequence, but in more limited ways.

We have previously described emotion as a shift in biasing of a number of body homeostatic systems, usually via hormones in the bloodstream. In short, we prepare for a different kind of activity by changing the settings—biases—of our many homeostatic systems. This kind of preparation also involves, of course, motor changes, as when a wild animal bares his fangs or the domestic cat arches its back when a dog threatens. As always, there is the inhibitory opposite: defeat or discouragement may produce a lowering rather than raising of biases. We droop, or cringe; an observer might say we look "crushed." What we mean by emotion is simply a generalized *preparation*, by adjusting biases, for a different kind of activity that we perceive may be required. When we climb stairs our heart beats faster in response to demand—that is not emotion. The sequence is wrong. Emotion typically occurs before the action, which in fact may not be put into effect if actual need for it does not develop.

At this point it may be helpful to examine Figure 13 and to trace step by step the processes going on. Let us assume a very early fish-like ancestor with a simple brain. (Even so, much of the circuitry is omitted in the diagram for the sake of clarity.)

The subject creature is already in a situation, since we flow from one situation into the next with no way of ever *not* being in a situation. Assume in this case that the fish is feeding, ingesting small particles of food as it hovers over a weed patch. The many aspects of this whole situation we will simply summarize as circle A.

At B we will deal with just one receptor, an eye—by no means as good an eye as humans have, but far more primitive both in itself and in terms of the recognition prosters it feeds to.

Since the creature has a brain, it is aggressive in probing its environment, which is to say it takes the initiative, and looks as well as sees. The dotted lines (1) represent looking, the solid line (2) the visual input falling on its retina as a result. This input derives from a dark object (C) some distance away and nearer the surface of the water.

From the visual receptor (B) binary-coded signals are routed to a perception proster, as shown by the line (3). Our creature does not have much brain, so its prosters are few and not well stocked with programs. In this instance the best recognition that can be matched is the stored program (4) which tentatively identifies the object as "possible predator."

Now follow the output (5) from this perception proster as it goes to an evaluation or main decision-making proster. Note that this proster has bias inputs from "Situation" A; and so biased, it selects from available alternative general programs the one marked (6) —namely, "leave" the scene because of "possible predator." If the subject creature had not eaten for a long time and was very hungry, the bias input marked "hunger" might have a stronger value and the

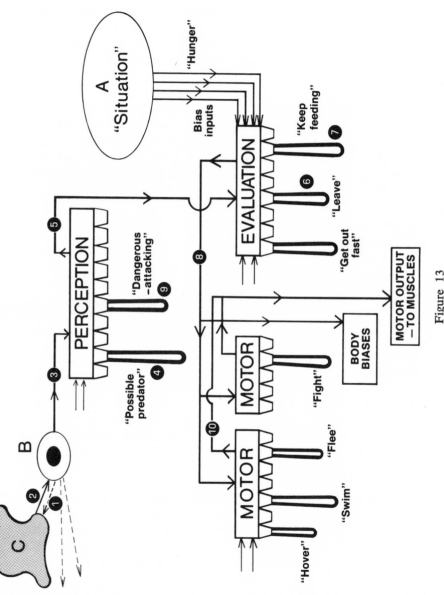

A
"Situation"

"Hunger"

Bias
inputs

EVALUATION

"Keep
feeding"
7

"Leave"
6

"Get out
fast"

B

PERCEPTION

5

"Dangerous
–attacking"
9

"Possible
predator"
4

3

8

MOTOR

"Fight"

BODY
BIASES

MOTOR OUTPUT
–TO MUSCLES

MOTOR

"Hover"

"Swim"

"Flee"

10

C

1
2

Figure 13

evaluation proster might instead switch on general program (7), be cautious but "keep on feeding." Let us assume that it has fed for awhile and that the "hunger" bias is therefore weak, and so (6) is put into effect.

The output from the evaluation proster, line (8), carries to the motor proster. For simplicity, we will assume here a choice exists of only three programs: "hover" as in feeding, "swim" as in normal locomotion, "flee" as in emergency. Closely linked is a "fight" proster which can be switched on by the higher-level evaluation proster if "flee" is perceived to be inadequate. Most animals will fight as a last resort, whatever the odds, if the circumstances permit. These prosters of course are being biased by many inputs (omitted in the diagram) from the situation as it changes from moment to moment. At this instant, "fight" stays switched off, and "hover" is now switched off and "swim" switched on, thus effecting in motor terms the evaluation decision to leave the scene.

Our subject starts swimming away at normal speed. Where it swims is a choice made by other prosters. But before long the continued radarlike probing and questioning of the environment by the eye results in a new clue being obtained: the behavior and shape of the dark mass is now identified by a recognition program (9) in the perception proster as "dangerous predator attacking."

A new perception signal now goes to the evaluation proster, which makes the decision "get out of here, fast!" New biases now affect the motor proster—"swim" is switched off and program "flee" is selected. Motor output signals are sent (10) to reach the muscles. Our creature now swims away at maximum speed.

But "flee" requires that the body biases that serve well enough for "swim" be reset. Energy must be released faster. Digestion can be stopped temporarily. By linkages too complex to show in this diagram, the housekeeping parts of the brain effect these shifts of body biases.

Let us say our subject is now chased against some rocks so that "flee" is aborted, and for lack of other alternative "fight" is switched on. This calls for further resetting of the body biases, for the animal may as well exhaust itself fighting as die by being eaten. The biases then are set at extremes, using energy at a pace that can be maintained only briefly.

What we mean by emotions (at least within Proster Theory) is this *resetting* of body biases. But such resetting is ordered by the brain; and accordingly the linkages involved in producing the orders cannot meaningfully be separated from the bias shifts themselves. If a judge orders a suspect to be put in jail, and he is, we cannot say sensibly that the judge is responsible for the order but not the jailing, or responsible for the jailing but not the order. Nor can we separate the brain's giving orders to reset body biases and the actual resetting. We may, of course, reset biases for "flee" but then countermand the order to flee; but the fact that we did not use the resetting does not change the fact that the resetting was accomplished. It is the resetting of biases, the preparation for a change in activity, that constitutes emotion. And the emotion involves the human brain at all levels. To oversimplify, the oldest brain does the body resetting, the middle brain gives the orders, and the new brain provides complex and detailed analysis of the situation and gives permission for or inhibits the emotion. But the new brain, the cerebral cortex and its associated pathways, does not always win. It can be temporarily shunted out of the decision making as older, simpler circuits take over. A suitable term for this is "downshifting."

Why and when does downshifting occur?

Again we must remember that the kind of brain we have reflects what happened to our phylogenetic line over hundreds of millions of years. During all but the last tiny fragment of that period, the first necessity of "brain" was that it provide for survival in simple physical terms. In our civilized daily existence, our ability directly to affect our survival has become blurred. The win-or-lose struggle that characterizes so much of nature has been transmuted to infinite gradations and complexities. We no longer live with death, aware that a predator may strike at any moment, that we must take frequent risk of death to gain the food to survive, that the coming of winter raises realistic doubts whether we shall again see the coming of spring. On the contrary, we assume that we shall live to seventy or more. The threats to long life take on an accidental, capricious quality: a heart attack out of the blue, an auto or airplane crash, an explosion, a flood, an earthquake. Or war, subjecting us to the sudden, unseen hazard of the bullet or mine or bomb that finds its mark.

We have little sense of control over these matters. They happen. As with losers at a roulette table, the wrong numbers came up.

Further, survival itself has become less a matter of live-or-die than one of existence graduated along many scales. The electricity fails, our house grows cold, the appliances won't operate, the television stays blank. Events beyond our influence, or even knowledge, have abruptly changed our level of existence. The same shift occurs when we lose employment because of a merger or are injured in an accident, or, in the other direction, are cured of a disease or inherit a fortune. Since we expect to live, *how* we live—by many criteria— becomes our focus, not simply "to be or not to be," which we often can't influence anyway.

But against these new attitudes and needs stands the great bulk of our life history in species terms, in terms of the thread of existence that stretches back half a billion years or longer. During most of these vast periods, the focus was on moment-to-moment and short-term survival. Our reptilian brain is still constructed primarily to meet that need. Our old mammalian brain, though far more elaborate and much more subtle in discerning situation, still operates by essentially the same rules—as it were, a few brief maxims that served at the reptilian stage have become several pages of sentences with "if" and "but" scattered liberally throughout. By comparison, the more recent neocortex is the reference room of a sizable library. It is not the place to go for a quick, simple, time-tested answer. There is too much information, too much variation and qualification, too much that gets in the way of an instantaneous decision on which survival itself may depend.

Two main factors operate here: speed and complexity.

To grasp the importance of the first, we can closely observe some sport—baseball will serve nicely. One appeal of the game no doubt stems from the yes/no simplifications it produces. A pitch is a strike or a ball, nothing between; a runner is either safe or out; a run either scores or it doesn't. At first base the call often hinges on ball or runner getting there as little as a tenth of a second earlier. The third baseman can catch a line smash if he gets his glove up in time, but if he reacts a split second slower, the ball goes into the outfield. In just this way, some ancestors of man survived if they dodged or hid, became a meal if they didn't, with the smallest fraction of time determining the result.

In other circumstances, especially where the distance between ancestor and possible aggressor was rapidly closing, a somewhat longer period of decision might exist, as in the instance diagrammed with the fishlike creature. In many animals this time factor creates a trigger distance: two dogs, for example, who might come together slowly without conflict may, if they surprise each other only a few feet apart, immediately attack. Big-game hunters know the dangers of getting within the trigger zone in deep grass or other concealment. In such instances the decision probably is being made at the reptilian level—the mammal downshifts. Time does not permit back-and-forth questioning of the environment and a search of recognition prosters; *to be wrong is to die* is the ancestral rule, expressed as "if there is no time to think, attack. Or if attack is impossible, flee."[4]

Thinking takes time. The computer vividly illustrates this: although individual electronic switching proceeds so rapidly that processing is measured in millionths of a second, a computing task may still take a computer minutes or even hours if sufficiently complex. In our bodies, moreover, systemic biasing involves a lag as hormones are carried to various parts of the body by the bloodstream. While we can act by muscle orders before the hormones take effect—as when we leap for the curb to escape an approaching car that surprises us—the hormones (the word derives from the Greek for "urge") are needed to maintain exceptional effort.

As any Little League coach knows, ballplayers must learn to evaluate the situation *before* a play occurs. A shortstop has no time to reflect on which base to throw to as he makes a stop—he has to execute a previous decision. Similarly, the skillful automobile driver decides to execute a left turn as soon as a certain approaching car passes, and does so, in contrast to the less able driver who lets the car pass, then decides—and finds another car is now bearing down, making the turn too risky. But we can make these advance decisions only in rather standardized settings, where they occur again and again. In Proster Theory terms, we build, by learning, a repertoire of programs, grouped (for baseball) as "two out," "bases loaded," "bunt likely," and other situational prosters—greatly shortening the recognition-decision-motor circuitry.

But obviously we cannot build and stock such short-cut prosters to cope with infrequent, surprising, or hard-to-recognize situations. Though the vast majority of these imply no threat to survival in a live-or-die sense, they nevertheless produce biasing, as evidenced in blushing, a flare of anger, change in breathing, tensing of muscles, dry throat, rising voice, tightening of "stomach," and so on.

Why should this be? Since the touchstone of this discussion is need, why do we have a gamut and variety of emotions? The reader may find this a reasonably acceptable scale, for example, in one continuum:

> Displeasure
> Irritation
> Annoyance
> Anger
> Rage
> Rage with aggression
> Violent rage with attack

What utility lies in biasing to the degree called for by irritation or anger? We can ask the same question of many emotions.

The answer, or at least a good part of it, brings us back to *signaling*. We are highly social creatures, and have been for a long time. *Social* always implies crowding, living in groups close together. This creates the constant need to signal to one another—the less that distance between individuals serves as a cushion or buffer to prevent sudden attack, the greater the necessity for the continual exchange of assurances of our intentions, mood, and relationships. To the postures, tensions, movements, and vocalizations animals use, humans add the enormous resources of speech—which has led us to neglect the nonverbal aspects, or signals. Biasing puts signals into speech: we speak of a cold or warm tone of voice, or of shrill anger or deep-throated rage.

We can watch signaling, formalized to a large degree, by observing automobile traffic. The intentions of the approaching driver became evident by his turn signals, the angle of his front wheels, choice of lane, change in speed, and so forth. The sight of a car that comes too fast or too slowly, or that wavers or gets where it shouldn't be, alarms us. By and large, the movement of thousands of vehicles on intersecting paths, as in the center of a city, is feasible only because of the constant sending of signals. Even the driver who proceeds down his proper lane is signaling "I am abiding by the rules," just as one who rashly cuts in is giving the opposite message. When the message is sent too late or isn't clear, a crash is likely.

When we are with other people we almost constantly signal and receive signals, or promptly feel distress, anxiety, or alarm. In an airplane or a doctor's waiting room we can encourage others to open conversation with us, or discourage them, by the signals we emit— here, as in perception, there can be a back-and-forth procedure in which questions are asked and more answers obtained, with or without the use of words.

Though the topic invites pursuit, adequate discussion lies beyond the scope of this book. That we rely heavily on signals is, I believe, obvious and not in serious question. Even within the field of public education, where talk reigns, there is now awareness of the importance of nonverbal signals, at least in some quarters.[5]

The second factor mentioned above, complexity, relates to speed in quantitative ways: the less circuitry involved, the faster the processing can be. But that is not the whole story. The limbic area, the old mammalian brain, has a crudity that sharply contrasts with the sophistication of the neomammalian gray matter. The elaborate, subtle new brain perceives and evaluates, but then has to pass its findings over to the severely limited middle brain that, with the assistance of a still more primitive reptilian brain, effects the body biasing.

MacLean, whose profound scholarship does not interfere with his colorful phraseology, some years ago wrote:

> Speaking allegorically of these three brains within a brain, we might imagine that when the psychiatrist bids the patient to lie on the couch, he is asking him to stretch out alongside a horse and a crocodile.[6]

Human, horse, and crocodile coexist inseparably in the structure of our brain. When we deal with people in the hope of influencing their behavior, or producing learning, we inescapably deal with this extraordinarily improbable Siamese triplet. How we deal with people, how they individually perceive and respond to situations, indeed how they use their own brains depend on the internal relations among the three kinds of brain.

The frequent and widespread use of the words "cognitive" and "affective" as essentially different and opposed ways of thinking—as thinking as opposed to feeling—muddies the waters and prevents understanding of what actually happens. This terminology derives in unbroken line from the eighteenth-century concept of soul as divided into three parts and functions: cognitive (thought), connative (will), and affective (feeling). It is not too soon, perhaps, to dump these vague, romantic terms in favor of something more closely related to the physical structures within our cranium. The key point is that we do not and cannot use one part of our brain rather than another, but that all the parts are intricately linked and have no independent existence or function.

CHAPTER 15

Threat, Risk, and Downshifting

WHAT I have termed downshifting means any emotional biasing away from the fullest use of the neocortex and its resources toward more reliance on older, cruder portions of the whole brain system.

In terms of speed, downshifting brings into use faster ways of making decisions. In earlier stages of our evolution, we were probably small mammals who moved around more than many, took more risks, faced more quick life-and-death decisions, all of which put a survival premium on the ability to throw the switches extremely rapidly. This way of life tended to produce more gray matter as generations passed. So the conflict between having and using all available brain, and downshifting to use only a part, but faster, got its start millions of years ago. Today's field mouse illustrates the point: perceiving some object dropping toward it, it can't afford to wait to determine nicely whether or not it is a hawk. Delay could be fatal. The same applies to complexity. The mouse cannot afford a mental debate as to which of several holes will serve best to hide in or what other evasive tactic might work. Traditional behavior has a virtue not always publicly examined, especially by traditionalists— it shortcuts thinking. You do what you did last time. In fact, you regularly prepare to do the usual, by having standard operating procedures, which is to say a standby proster ready to put into effect the often-used programs, varied only as conditions demand. We can feel sure that the field mouse, no less than the ballplayer, makes decisions in advance. By an established program, it continually notes where the nearest hiding place is, so no time will be lost thinking should the hawk threat appear. If its caution proves to be unwarranted, the mouse can resume its previous activity with no more than a small loss of time and energy.

But note what happened. The mouse cut off its normal clueing process, the back-and-forth obtaining of first clues, asking for more for confirmation, finally finding a match in a recognition proster. At the first crude perception of threat, the creature downshifts and takes traditional action.

We are no longer mice escaping swift predators. Our sense of threat has become graded over a wide continuum. But the principle remains: under threat, we downshift to cruder, more traditional (either for the individual or species, or both) ways of behaving.

For analogy, picture the owner of a yacht who permits his teenage son to take the helm on many occasions, but who in a storm, or entering a tricky channel, hovers over the youth with evident lack of confidence, and at the sign of further danger pushes him aside and takes the wheel himself. Perhaps he acknowledges that the lad may know more technically about operating the boat and its electronic gear than he does, but the older man puts more trust in his experience. He has survived a thousand voyages, the youngster only dozens; he has met emergencies by trusting his eyes and the feel of the boat rather than the radio compass. This differing view of abilities may cause bickering, but in the face of threat the father feels justified in taking over abruptly.

The degree of downshifting will roughly be proportionate to the degree of threat perceived—perceived, as before, meaning by the individual. There will also be a generalized bias: the less secure or confident the individual, the more readily threat will be perceived, and the faster and deeper the downshifting.

We see this dramatically revealed in emergencies. Our car crashes into another. We may feel fear or rage, and later find that we have available singularly little detail about what happened—and make very poor witnesses. "It all happened so fast," we explain. What we actually experienced was a sharp downshift under severe stress. The elaborate back-and-forth process of perception was so thoroughly cut off that we have to struggle to reconstruct even elementary facts.

Similarly, a person deeply offended in public may be unable to make any spoken response, though later brilliant rejoinders readily come to mind.

Under threat we downshift. Under *sudden* threat the downshift may cut off even evaluating the threat, so we downshift all the more, resorting to a few traditional behaviors: run, fight, seek the comfort of a group, or the security of home or a substitute shelter. If none of these seem possible, most likely we stand rooted to the ground, even if clearly we have more sophisticated but less often used prosters to choose from. Commonly, we also temporarily lose the power of speech—one of the newest brain functions—and at best can make only some kind of noise. In his *Textbook of Psychology*, Hebb states:

> Though we ordinarily think of emotional excitement as a cause of vigorous, effective response—that is, we think of it as motivating— there is well-authenticated evidence showing not only that it can impair behavior but also that it can reduce the effectiveness of response to near zero . . . in extreme cases, the subject's thought may be so impaired that he really does not have what we would ordinarily consider to be fear or terror.[1]

Hebb notes other studies of behavior in disasters such as fires or flash floods which show that few people manage organized behavior appropriate to the emergency, and still other studies of infantrymen in battle agree that only a small percentage can be relied on to aim and fire their weapons.

Studies of people's behavior in less sudden emergencies, such as an approaching flood or tornado, show plainly that they do not rush wildly about or behave in new ways. On the contrary, they often persist in staying put in their homes, or calmly follow some well-established prosters that take them to friends or relatives or on some other familiar pathway. Under severe stress, we are typically least capable of using new or infrequent behaviors quickly, although given a good deal of time we may at length improvise. Downshifting is always to more traditional, more familiar, cruder behavior—to what we would do if we had much less brain.

Sudden emergencies serve to tell us a good deal about the security individuals feel, at least under that particular kind of threat. At the cry of "fire!" some may go to pieces and need to be virtually pushed out of the building, while others calmly take conventional action. Ordinarily, the individual's ability to cope with a variety of threat reflects a general level of self-confidence.

Under milder threat, the downshift may take a more limited form of shortening the back-and-forth process of perception input and matching. We can call this "irising," in the sense of the iris of a camera lens or of the eye shutting down so that less light enters. We perceive less, and even that not so sharply, so that in effect much less input is acquired. It's as though the nervous middle brain were telling the new brain, "Hurry up, hurry up, we can't risk all that time!" Every classroom teacher has seen the effect on children: they stab at answers, guess wildly, garble, miss even gross distinctions. Most executives have seen a little-experienced secretary respond the same way to pressure, irising down so that instructions either don't register at all or are misunderstood. Nor is the executive exempt under comparable circumstances.

When we look at children called (absurdly) "minimally brain damaged" (or any of the many equivalent terms), the same response seems evident in exaggerated form. Proster Theory would suggest that most of these children feel so constantly under threat that the perception process becomes severely abbreviated. They observe soon enough that their perceptions do not seem to be reliable or accepted by others around them, and this creates more threat. It may well be that there is nothing wrong with their brains, but a lot wrong with their experience.

I will not attempt any profound analysis of threat. Perhaps others will, or have done work that could be applied in this context. What is clear, however, is that downshifting and irising are exceedingly common and familiar in individual experience and observation. Further, we can distinguish various levels.

The most abrupt and vigorous downshift involves threat to our creature existence: we are faced with possible death. Only slightly less intense is the prospect of serious pain, injury, maiming, or disfigurement. At the lowest level we seek to avoid temporary discomfort. Phylogenetically, these are the oldest forms of threat.

There also appear to be two important social categories of threat. One derives from the helplessness of the human infant—many years pass before the child can care for himself and escape hazards on his own. Separation from parental care carries threat in varying degrees. In infancy, even a week's separation from the mother can have traumatic long-term effects. And as man is a social animal, descended from social animals, there is likely a deep-seated fear throughout life of not being part of a group, not being "in" and thus protected and accepted. This involves status, pecking order, and group role. Second, man uniquely acquires possessions that become interwoven with status, acceptance, and security. On yet another but related plane, man utilizes symbols, which, in turn, carry with them a sense of both past and future. Threat, which initially concerned only the present and stressed instant action, can be converted by man's complex brain into anxiety, oriented toward future and lacking the sharp focus of survival threat. Anxiety is typically diffuse, even "nameless"—as in Leviticus: "Ye shall flee when none pursueth you."

One other type of threat must be noted: confinement. Even the puniest creature when cornered may, as a last resort, turn on a far superior aggressor. From far back in our history comes the idea of freedom to move as offering escape and possible survival, and of lack of running room as signifying early doom. Though the infant will accept being held firmly by a parent or familiar person, the stranger who holds the baby the same way can expect a vigorous outcry. Some months later, grasping or confining the child usually will provoke screams and struggle. Should you be locked in the comfortable, familiar room where you may be reading a book, you would probably find yourself merely by that knowledge distressed and unable to concentrate. We regard confinement *in itself* as being punishment: consider stocks or pillory; prison; in school, "detention"; with small children, "stand in the corner."

For present purposes, then, threat can be seen as anything perceived by the individual as presenting the hazard of bodily damage, separation from protectors, lowering of group status (to the ultimate of exclusion), damage to possessions or symbols, or confinement in some form.

The presence of threat in any of these five forms (there may well be more) or in combinations, produces irising and downshifting in more or less corresponding degree. In plainest language, if we wish people to use the enormous power of their new, human brain, as distinct from the middle and oldest brains, we have to put them in circumstances in which threat is absent.

It is hardly possible to miss the astounding unsuitability of schools on this count. With rare exception, the school confines its students, first to an institutional building, then to a specific four-walled room, for twelve years or so, with no chance even of time off for good behavior. In many schools, physical punishment—beating—is still permitted. Other serious punishments are expulsion or suspension—separation in purest form, a devastating threat. Within the ordinary classroom, reprimand, sarcasm, put-down, publicly exposed and recorded failure, and the laughter, mockery, or rejection of class-mates are never more than a second away. Those who bring posses-sions and symbols, including the language of their home, that do not conform to the teacher's idea of middle-class norm may suffer fre-quent and serious abuse. Throughout, the student is systematically separated from protectors and left in the hands of dictators given powers found nowhere else in our society. The kindliest teacher represents threat, for the power is always available. That most schools aggressively crush thinking can hardly be wondered at. That we spend billions on such schools and compel children to attend, can be.

We need to distinguish, of course, between threat, which is im-posed from without—often with sudden peaks—and the deliberate acceptance of *risk*: as with the little girl who insists on walking a plank across a ditch, the teenager who tries drugs *because* they are dangerous, the housewife who plays the horses, and the businessman who speculates in volatile securities. Threatened, a child scowls, cries, runs. Allowed to take such risk as it wishes, it grins and evinces pleasure. Willingness to assume risk, apart from neurotic motives of punishing self or parent, gives a good measure of inner security. The healthy, growing child—and to a lesser degree the adult, until age brings decline—wants risk, seeks it actively, must have it. Risk is to thinking as vitamins are to nourishment.

The phenomena I have called downshifting and irising have re-ceived little rigorous attention and study.[2] To be sure, downshifting can be understood only if one has some grasp of how the human brain evolved and is constructed, and irising only if one views per-ception as a continuing, back-and-forth, radarlike process that can be cut short. Neither of these concepts has been widely popular, although both are far from new; the combination has had still less attention.

Yet, once we understand these concepts and the apparatus they involve, we can observe the phenomena exhibited daily in others, and in ourselves. This hardly constitutes scientific evidence; but we are concerned here with developing theory rather than substantive bits of proof, which may be developed in due course, or which may exist, camouflaged by other contexts and terminologies. And I hope these concepts begin to suggest what we should do to create conditions that foster the kind of thought, learning, and behavior we need to survive in today's world.

CHAPTER 16

Thinking the Natural Way—
Or the Hard Way

Harvey and Henry, their sixth-grade teacher will tell you, are hopeless in mathematics. They have not mastered the simplest elements of arithmetic.

But when the two boys escape to the playground, Harvey can throw a high fly to Henry some two hundred feet away, and Henry, after watching the ball's flight for a second or two, can move almost exactly to where the ball will fall.

How can these boys, so "stupid" in arithmetic inside the classroom, somehow when outside solve in seconds the complicated equations that predict precisely where the ball will drop—taking into consideration the initial velocity and inclination, deceleration and acceleration of gravity, air resistance, windage, curve due to rotation, and slope of the ground?

The physical act of catching the ball involves the selection of a combination of motor programs from a complex "catching a ball" hierarchy. But that does not help answer the "where" question. And obviously no two throws ever follow quite the same trajectory, so the solution cannot simply be pulled out of memory. Rather the answer is found by remarkable differential analysis, the glory of this thirty-billion-plus-neuron brain. A back-and-forth process of perception is going on; the situation is being compiled by simultaneous search of untold recognition prosters, with crosschecking and comparative analysis leading to a decision. The teacher may protest, "This is not mathematics!" True, no symbols were selected and then manipulated—but the boy caught the ball. Should a throw be high, Henry may even launch himself into the air so that the path of his rising hand precisely intercepts the constantly curving flight of the ball, a feat that more than doubles the complexity of the solution needed. Something went on in the "arithmetic-stupid" brain that solved the problem. Whatever we call it, it would seem pretty useful, and deserving of respect.

In recent years, it seems to me, greater acceptance has developed of what may be called intuitive or heuristic modes of thought. Still, practically everyone has to go through long years of formal education, and most better jobs require certain credentials, awarded primarily for conforming to whatever the educational institutions may demand. As a result we all tend to suffer from the most stupendous, organized, incessant brainwashing of all: the obsession formal education has with rational and logical processes, heavily dependent on verbalization. But suppose we could by some magical means strip away from our sciences and technologies and practical arts all that did *not* spring from rational and logical manipulation of symbols: all the accidental discoveries, the instances of serendipity, the products of hunches and ideas that "pop into the head out of nowhere," all the endless adaptations and combinations of previous patterns, all the motor skills, the gradually built techniques, the trial and error . . . we would be early hominids, with the invention of the wheel ages in the future. Rational and logical thinking did produce most of the stubborn *wrong* answers that beset the world and frustrated man for centuries. Most of scientific history records a struggle against logical, rational ideas: the scientific age began when we stopped thinking in those ways and began observing, measuring, and "dreaming up" theory to be tested.

Yet in schools and colleges and throughout much of adult life, rational, logical, symbolized, and verbalized modes of thought are worshipped; and basic, natural thinking is despised, even punished.

The great bulk of human brainpower suffers suppression and disparagement because of this witless, pompous, pretentious emphasis on largely nonproductive but respectable artificial modes of thought, kept dominant with reptilian tenacity. If Harvey and Henry can correctly add 14 and 11 and 8 and divide the sum by 3, using approved algorithms, they win praise. That in catching the ball they solve problems that would take an analog computer considerable time to program and read out, or give a large digital unit a long workout, counts for nothing! The sad fact that classical and horsesense logic almost always produce wrong answers could hardly be more evident. (The newer logics that do have specialized productivity in skilled hands are known to few persons.)

It is hardly too much to say, as a working rule, that anything that sounds logical in the usual sense can be assumed to be wrong, because it is *too simple*. As we have over millennia learned more about the world we inhabit, and ourselves, we have consistently opened up new levels of complexities. Magic is simpler than science, folklore simpler than reality. The more a science advances, the more "incredible" its findings become.

If conventional logic is worse than useless, symbols do have enormous and critically human usefulness for recording and communication. Only by employing symbols can we accumulate and pass on our great store of knowledge and ideas. But for thinking, symbols prove clumsy, slow, and unreliable. Two severe handicaps immediately appear. The first is that conventional symbolic thought proceeds sequentially, along a single line—but as we have seen, the human brain has enormous capability to handle simultaneous processing, not necessarily in any logical sequence at all. The second is that if the sequential effort should be defective or ambiguous at any point, the consequences of error multiply. For example, if someone giving you directions advises you to "drive to the bridge, turn right for a half-mile, then left for five traffic lights, and next right for a mile," one left instead of right or one missed point will put you miles away from your objective. But the natural kind of information processing that goes on in the brain is differential and comparative, which to say that it is self-checking. In addition, it makes constant use of feedback. As a result it is infinitely faster, more exhaustive, and more reliable.

We can identify two opposing modes of thinking, at either end of a continuum, since blending is possible. We can designate rational or "respectable" thinking as SSM (for symbol selection and manipulation). The natural, proster type of thinking we can call PAC (for perception, analysis, choice). PAC can be said to be subconscious or subrational or may be called intuitive, but all these terms raise problems of connotations that we can avoid by using PAC and SSM.

As we have seen, the brain directs what we call attention or conscious effort to primarily one matter at a time. The abortion of a program interrupts, because inability to carry out a selected program means one of two things: either the decision to select and implement that program was faulty, or some change in circumstances has occurred that demands reevaluation. In general, perception of new or added threat in the situation has the same effect; it interrupts, takes precedence, for evident survival reasons.

At the SSM end of the continuum, symbol manipulation requires a high degree of attention, unless the activity can be relegated to well-established prosters. For example, a figure clerk using an adding machine may be able to make hundreds of entries and even carry out a considerable program, taking totals and transferring, without full concentration on the operation. An illegible figure, a strange or incorrect document, a noise in the machine, or any change in the routine serves as an abortion and immediately commands full attention. It is this abortion mechanism that permits handling routines without full attention. But new tasks, strange elements, changes in the setting, or the introduction of threat demand that the activity come front and center. Inherently, then, SSM requires substantial effort, and exhibits a fragility of continuity: we have to work hard at keeping our attention on the effort, and so we often set up favorable conditions such as a quiet room, minimum movement, and comfortable, secure conditions. (Classrooms, typically, are noisy, full of movement, often uncomfortable, and drenched in threat. We now know that even the less threatening "open" school needs to provide dividers, carrels, and small spaces. Not a few offices and shops where SSM is called for offer similar handicaps. "It's so hectic here I can't think," an employee may say.)

Some years ago a circus performer attracted star billing and notice for his feat of standing on one finger. SSM at an extreme appears to be the mental equivalent. A huge load is placed on that one small function of the brain that can be brought into the attention zone for a period. The feat is possible, like the circus act, but it seems more sensible to stand on the large-muscled legs and to use the full resources of our glorious neocortex. PAC *uses* the multibillion-neuron capacity of the brain, while SSM hobbles it and puts obstacles and booby traps in the way. If we observe large quantities of new-task SSM effort, as in almost any common form of examination (excluding some multiple-choice) given to children or adults, we find a huge proportion of wrong answers. Schools, colleges, government agencies, businesses, and other formal institutions dote on SSM because it can be written down, standardized, examined, graded, counted. It is relatively simple, and it has great appeal to functionaries who must deal with such complex entities as people, or involved technical, business, economic, or political problems, and who yearn for *something* to be simple. And for teachers at any level, SSM has a welcome visibility. The student who arrives at answers or solutions—but cannot explain how—annoys or frightens the teacher; the executive who cannot provide a neat rationale for a program he or she has thought out will have trouble getting approval. Fortunately, most creative and productive people soon learn to find solutions by PAC and then convert the results into respectable SSM terms. But only the bolder individuals defy convention by openly disparaging the "logic" and "orderly thinking" that is officially admired so universally. Not a few people, we may guess, succeed in brainwashing themselves—particularly those with strong guilt feelings who cannot tolerate the notion of effortless thinking producing good or even great results.

But the PAC mode of thinking, though it uses much body energy, essentially *is* effortless. The work aspect lies in providing the brain with raw input, as in observing, reading, collecting data, and reviewing what others have achieved. Once in, PAC procedures take over, simultaneously, automatically, outside of the attention zone—provided threat does not produce downshifting and halt or suspend the operation. Typically, there is no way to effect the input logically or sequentially, any more than a builder can order his materials before he has his design. Nor does it much matter whether the builder first gives attention to bricks or beams or plaster: at this stage he cannot know what he will require nor in what order it must be delivered, or what interactions will have importance. PAC thinking begins with utter disorder and a random, fortuitous approach. Order emerges as the *result*. But the vast majority of people in any way instructing others generally, in deference to the SSM convention, try to foist order and sequence on the learner—try to start the student where the instructor has ended.

SSM has its place, as I have suggested. But the vast bulk of useful, productive, creative thinking or switch-throwing that goes on in the human brain falls dominantly into the PAC category. When we discourage PAC, when we persistently tell people that only SSM is respectable, we cripple the use of the human brain to the extent that they believe it. The great ally of SSM is formal education, at all levels; it is, conversely, the great enemy of PAC. Nor am I the first to hint that education makes many people stupid.

A fascinating aspect of the PAC mode, at that extreme end of the continuum, is what I call search.

One would have to look far to find any person noted for creative or problem-solving work who cannot testify from repeated personal experiences that PAC is not only capable of almost instantaneous achievements but also of long-continuing effort. Given a problem and the necessary raw inputs, and "left alone" to deal with it, our neocortex obligingly will solve it and serve the answers up neatly in due course.

Scientists and inventors, for example, have related again and again how the answers to problems they were struggling to find suddenly "popped into the head" hours or days after they had, by concentrating on input, inserted the problem into the brain as one might feed a computer. The patterns are familiar: the individual suddenly wakes up with the solution, or as in the classic instance of Archimedes, finds the answer prompted by some seemingly unrelated activity—in his case taking a bath.

I am fully convinced that use of PAC can be deliberately encouraged. For years, in solving my own creative problems, I have declined to "work" on them, but instead have inserted the input, as one puts laundry into a washer and confidently pushes the starting button. In good time, the answers almost always arrive, although the more intricate the problem and complex the input, the longer the solution may take.

Nathan observes in this connection: "Strange as it may seem, creation comes from pouring a great mass of ill-assorted things into the mind, leaving them to ferment, and then getting something new out of it."[1] He further notes that much must be put in, with intense concentration as a rule, for the creative output to be achieved. One might say that the answer comes easily, but the question takes effort.

It seems apparent (since obviously many creative people work this way) that a search is going on during the interval, though not necessarily continuously—much as in a large computer. I would hazard the guess that the search ramifies, starts and stops, reaches dead ends and begins afresh, and eventually assembles an answer that is evaluated and then popped into conscious attention—often in astonishingly full-blown detail. As a rule, it seems, the answer can get through only when no threat or great amount of SSM is in the way. PAC answers characteristically arrive in bed, while doing small chores or routine tasks, or during mild entertainment. The whole field of how to encourage PAC and thus really use the full facilities of the neocortex is so unexplored as to be almost frightening.

On a less exotic level, we commonly experience search when we find we cannot recall a name, a word, or some bit of information when we want it. Some time later, a few minutes or a few hours, the answer pops, when our attention is on other matters. The implication is strong that search has been going on during at least part of the interval, and a categorizing-down recall process has either become unblocked or has found an alternative pathway. Here again, quite simple techniques can greatly enhance recall ability, but the field has had little systematic study.

For their interest as examples, let me record two personal instances of referral to PAC mode, or "subattentional" thought.

Some months ago, a car registration form could not be found. Several persons in my family had handled it, and the trail was cold. I invited my neocortex to find it. A number of hours later it popped an answer: in my wallet. Of course I had already looked there— twice, in fact. Now I looked again, with care. No registration. This was baffling, because it has not been my experience that subattentional search produces wrong answers. (When a name or word you want to recall finally does pop, it is always the right one, as you may have observed.) Accordingly, I reinserted the request. The answer took over a day to come this time, but it was explicit: the form was in my wallet, and it was inside another form. I pulled the contents out, opening every folded piece of paper. Inside my Blue Cross identification was the registration.

The second instance began when I returned home late one pitch-black night, to be told by my wife that my neighbor had been out calling and searching for his old and clever dog, also pitch-black. It could not be found. Since I had not the vaguest idea where the animal might be—it was given to wandering about the neighborhood —I put my PAC apparatus in charge and moved into the woods behind our houses. Several minutes later, on a small path, I had an impulse to stop and flash my light toward the ground. A foot away from my left leg was the dog. Apparently it had ingested some bad food or water and was so bloated and almost paralyzed that it could neither walk nor make a sound. I carried the poor creature to its home, where happily it recovered. Possibly pure luck led me to that path and to stop right by the dog, but I would rather put my faith in thirty billion neurons allowed to work their own subtle way, combining all the information my brain had stored on the woods and the dog's behavior patterns.

These instances—and many readers, I am sure, can add their own and better—involve no magic or extrasensory perception, a term I find unfortunate.

We are far from understanding in detail what goes on in the neocortex, although the last twenty years have produced exciting leads. But the diagrammatic concept of prosters in hierarchies seems helpful. With enough prosters, enough kinds of prosters, enough interconnections, enough memory facilities, the thinking potential of our newest brain becomes staggering, and its miracles of performance less astonishing if no less remarkable. To cripple this magnificent instrument by pointless threat and SSM demands improperly applied is a crime against the very essence of human nature.

CHAPTER 17

The Use and Abuse of Words

$\mathbf{M}$AN, I am hardly the first to point out, is the "talking animal." Whether speech led to brain development or development to speech is an unanswered chicken-and-egg question; but certainly the complexity of the brain and the use of speech are not unrelated. Even the physical production of the noises we call speech involves a most intricate coordination of abdominal muscles, thorax, larynx, pharynx, tongue, lips, and to a degree cheeks. Air has to be precisely expelled, even as we continue to breathe for oxygen exchange. We not only produce the sounds, but vary tone and pitch, alter rhythm, change loudness and the "shape" of words—very likely adding gesture and facial expressions, even if we are talking over the telephone.[1] But all this is nothing compared to storing a vocabulary of tens of thousands of words, most of which we can call into use with only a fraction of a second delay, and the still largely baffling arrangement of these words into an order that gives them meaning to others with impressive subtlety and precision.

A considerable area of the cortex, almost always in the left hemisphere and, roughly speaking, behind the external ear, is vital to the use of speech. This should not be thought of as where speech "is," but as a main organizing and control area. As we have just noted, the process is most complex and involves many parts of the neocortex. For evolutionary reasons discussed in Part I, the brain attains intricate operations by elaborating older and simpler ones. The cries associated with the cruder emotions can all be produced, even by humans, without use of the neocortex. But speech is strictly a function of the newest brain; and when we downshift hard under threat the ability to speak is usually largely or entirely lost. A very scared, angry, or surprised person may not be able to get a word out. A thoroughly enraged one, as we often see, may be able to do no more than get out a few words, often expletives or abusive terms, which are repeated over and over. If a sentence is produced, it too is likely to be said again and again. Even a mild emotional shock can result in being "left speechless," stammering, and being restricted to a scant vocabulary. If we need familiar and dramatic evidence of downshifting, we can hardly find any better.

In the discussion of PAC and SSM modes, I did not mean to give any impression that words, being symbols, have no role in PAC, or are not "natural." Man does not merely learn to use speech; it is as built-in, as provided for in the blueprints, as walking upright. We are equipped with a speech-producing brain as an elephant is equipped with a trunk, and in addition, with elaborate word-sounding structures that other primates lack, that would be pointless without speech. Considerable evidence suggests that the left temporal lobe and adjacent areas so important to adult speech are at birth ordinarily "reserved" for this purpose—much as certain tables in a restaurant are held empty for guests expected to arrive later. The priority given speech functions appears to be exceedingly high; the brain will organize them elsewhere only if this left-side space has been severely damaged, and even then only in early childhood will it establish them at all well anywhere else.

We must say, then, that it is natural for this organizing area of cortex to think in words. That is what it is for. If we consider the right hemisphere, however, in roughly the corresponding location we find the organizing area for spatial concerns, including a sense of one's body as it fits into surrounding space. Normally development of this begins at infancy. In time it becomes the chief means by which a sculptor envisions a statue in the round, an engineer pictures a gear train, or an architect conceives a new massing. Most musical functions are also organized on this side, as are many aspects of mathematics.[2] There seems no compelling reason to suppose that the engineer, sculptor, architect, and musician don't think often in nonverbal terms, and much indication that they do. Those remarkable but not really rare individuals who can do very rapid mental mathematics—some faster than a mechanical calculator—obviously are using a nonverbal, "direct" method: their speed rules out symbol manipulation. Idiot savants, to use the old term for those who have this ability but little else, provide an excellent example: they usually are very inept at using symbols. In music, the self-taught or "natural ear" player or composer commonly doesn't know the symbols for what he or she is doing and can't explain how the often superb results are produced—apparently purest PAC.

Finally, we must consider animals. In view of their behavior and the clear fact that they have gray matter, we must agree that they think, yet since they have no speech they cannot think in words. (Chimpanzees have been proved able to learn and use quite a number of "words," provided they can use standard sign language such as deaf people "speak," or plastic shapes as written words. They seem to find such a vocabulary very handy.)[3]

We must conclude that thinking—which after all is simply the throwing of switches—does not rest exclusively on the use of words. On the other hand, we can see that words can be enormously useful in human thinking. While this subject can be no more than touched upon within the scope of this book, we can at least note some of the levels on which words can be used.

For sorting certain reference papers, I have an array of small drawers in different colors. The colors give no information about contents, but serve as markers. I can recall that a certain article is in the green drawer, or direct someone to look in the red one for something else. If the drawers were all white, I could achieve the same result by lettering on them "green," "red," "blue," and so on. We mark people this way by giving them names. Peter, Muriel, Harold, Joan are primarily markers; "primarily" because Angelo, Sven, and Ali are markers too, but these make apparent that in some circumstances a marker may carry information (here sex and ethnicity) as well. We need caution in ascertaining levels.

A restaurant door marked "men" gives more information than just the word. Here the word plainly serves as a clue, an identifier. The label "taxes," on one of my file drawers, goes further, for it suggests a classification of certain records out of many. My mail tray that says "answer" not only identifies and classifies, but effectively clues an elaborate proster.

Words can carry an astonishing amount of information. Suppose a husband who has been having hard times phones his wife and says, "I got a job." Or someone running by my front door calls, "The white house on the corner is on fire." If we examine language closely, however, we soon see that an astonishing amount of the information that the words seem to carry actually is not present except as the words serve as clues within the receiver's situation. Said to a stranger, "I got a job" could mean, in common usage, that the speaker is employed, that he has an assignment, or that he obtained employment at some unstated time and place, each of these a far cry from what the words meant to the wife. The nine short words about the fire enable me to picture exactly the house in question, the fact that it is old and wooden and could burn fast, the plight of the owners, both elderly and one in a wheelchair, and the fine paintings in the living room that I can visualize being destroyed. All of this has been clued by the few words that would tell a stranger merely that some house somewhere was on fire.

We tend to forget this in communicating by words. Even the person highly skilled in their use cannot know that some of the words used may be unintended clues to certain of his listeners—at any meeting we can see individuals hearing what was never explicitly said or meant. We also habitually put far too much importance on the words uttered, and too little on the nonverbal signals that go along with the spoken message and may or may not confirm it. On the speaker's side, too, error can readily enter because clues are assumed to be information-rich when they are not. Crude examples would be a lecturer's frequent mention of NATO when some hearers do not know what is referred to, or a teacher mentioning "sitting down to a meal" to children from families that don't ordinarily eat together. The teacher may have no awareness that the custom isn't universal.

How heavily ordinary speech depends on preexisting or situational knowledge can be perceived easily by simply going into some unfamiliar environment: a stockbrokers' office, a scientific laboratory, a convention, a place where some sport is in progress. Much of the talk heard will simply be meaningless. At a bowling match, for example, the nonbowler might hear:

"It never came up."
"He's on a turkey."
"Solid four."
"Nice cover!"
"I was clean for eight."

Most of the remarks by the players, in fact, might well be totally unintelligible to the neophyte in the audience. The problem is not simply that the words are unfamiliar, but that the comments have been stripped down to bare clues. If you cannot use the clues, you are baffled.

Worse, clues can mislead—more serious than gathering no meaning is getting the wrong meaning. If on hearing the remark about a turkey I infer that there is a bird as a prize or bet, I would be further off the track than before.[4] In the formal educational setting, particularly with younger students, this problem can become acute; the teacher dealing with thirty students who differ widely in background, experience, and previous input inevitably will use words that serve as false clues to certain members of the group. In arithmetic "carry," for instance, may mislead a student who has a vivid concept of that word, perhaps from having used it very early in life as a request to his parent to be picked up. He cannot interpret it as "transport" or "move to another place." Similarly, a student who clues "point" as the act of indicating with the finger and arm may have trouble seeing the term as "location" in geometry. When the teacher says, "We call this a point, and this line connects two points," the student distorts the meaning to see the line as "pointing" in two directions. For teachers to discover these false clues can be exceedingly difficult, especially since in typical classrooms teacher and student may never have a conversation that runs more than a few seconds, as observation with a stopwatch distressingly shows.

Words are enormously useful in thinking on the levels of markers, classifiers, and clues. But, I submit, we tend to vastly overestimate the *intrinsic* informational content of words, by attributing to these symbols meaning that actually resides in their situational use: the meaning is not in the word, but in when, where, how, and in what reference the word is used. This seems true both in the internal thinking process and in communication. When the effort is made to communicate or instruct with high dependence on the idea that words themselves have rich meaning, the result tends to have extremely low, or even negative, efficiency. Political campaigns illustrate the point all too well. Few voters at election time can state what the candidates have established verbally, even in elemental terms. Decisions rest far more on perceived nonverbal signals, on clues, and on markers. Since words may signify little, this is not necessarily regrettable.

Many have observed that talk is the most apparent curse of our educational system, and that teachers do the great bulk of the talking that goes on endlessly in conventional classrooms. Complaints about excess lecturing at the college level express the same fault; and in general our first tendency in trying to instruct anyone, for any purpose, is to talk at them. Since we talk for everyday communication mostly in situational mode, with high effectiveness, we slip all too easily into assuming that almost useless nonsituational talk will also work. (Only the highly trained, experienced, and skillful communicator has much sense of, or concern with, the difference between the two modes.)

The printed word presents the same broad problem: it serves to communicate primarily as it is situational—as it has markers and clues for the reader. A familiar and aggravating example can be the directions enclosed with some device that requires assembly after purchase. The engineer responsible instructs the reader to fit the clevis over the keyed end of the actuating rod, up to the flange, and then fasten it with the cotter pin. It is all amply situational to the engineer, and all pure Sanskrit to the consumer. We understand as much as we do of general written material because we each *select* what is likely to be situational and avoid what isn't. When a student does not have this privilege with textbooks, the value of the printed matter may drop very low, the more so if insistence is made on the use of one text rather than several.

To use speech in SSM style—tightly organized, precise, and rich in nonsituational meaning—requires considerable skill as well as confidence and experience, and we find very few people well qualified. To write nonsituationally takes a great deal more. Not surprisingly, we find that the great majority of persons called literate seldom write other than situationally, as in a note to the milkman, a letter to a friend, a memo to the boss, an order to a supplier. Or writing is done for purpose of record, which is also as a rule situational. The number of people who write more than very occasionally comes to an extremely small fraction of the human species. While only man writes, man can hardly be called the writing animal.

How do we recognize words? How do we pull them out of storage, arrange them in proper order, and utter them? The very complexity of this task provides a test of any model of brain operation.

Proster Theory suggests the main organization, though we cannot pursue its application to linguistics here. We can see each word as a program, arranged in prosters of related words of which only one will be selected at a time. The method of categorizing down presents a question: with fifty or seventy thousand words in storage, how can the incoming signal be matched with the stored program fast enough to understand speech?

We may note first that we do not recognize words instantly, but only after a perceptible lag. Often, after a missed word, we simply wait to get more context or some other clue, perhaps nonverbal, to what it was. Most speech is heavily redundant, and missing a good deal does not prevent catching the meaning—the more so if it is strongly situational. What occurs, apparently, is a pattern match: from those words we recognized and other clues we gathered, we project the pattern of what was not sharply heard. If the projection fits the heard pattern overall, we assume we are on track.[5] If the pattern does not fit, the effect is like that of a wrong meter in a poem, or a sour chord in a piece of music. It serves as an abortion, and so compels our attention, and if convenient we will ask for a repeat by the speaker.

If this were not so, the person with an enormous vocabulary would be slower to recognize words—there would be more searching necessary. We observe the contrary: the very skilled user of words seems to grasp meaning more rapidly than others. If context plays the dominant role, this would not be surprising. Context here means, however, not simply the words on either side, but the entire situation as perceived. If we are listening to a man whose face is flushed with anger and who is gesturing threateningly, we hardly expect he is telling us about his new grandson or reciting the latest grain-production estimates. A group standing around a large fish just hooked and landed are probably not discussing the value of an office building. Categorizing down, then, is likely primarily (and simultaneously) by setting, by subject, by situation, and by *expected* sequitur. There is not merely one storage point for often-used words, but many; the same word occurs in a number of prosters, each organized on the basis of different relationships. For example, "deck" is associated with playing cards and game setting, and with boats and boating. Though many words have several meanings, we usually have no trouble grasping the correct one, because the many clues available have directed search to the right proster.

This arrangement also may throw light on why we can recognize what is being said fairly easily, even when the speaker pronounces the words in a far from standard way. We have trouble with strange dialects or foreign accents mainly when both signals and situational factors are also unfamiliar. Or these may be lacking, as in a phone call from a stranger. If you do not regularly listen to popular music, try learning the lyrics of a rock group's song! Via record or radio, we may require many hearings to catch even a few words, without much in signals or situational factors to help.

We can find words, no doubt, by pure phonetic, one-track categorizing down—the method used to deliver the mail, using only an address of syllables. But this is the hard, slow way, a sort of last resort backup for the quick way: recognition achieved by use of the several methods simultaneously, with syntax pattern confirming recognition based on sometimes skimpy clues.

Stored programs need not be limited to one syllable or a single word. Much of our speech consists of frequently used combinations, up to and including the "recordings" many individuals annoy us with, to retell an incident, register a complaint, express frozen prejudices, or bridge a social lacuna with small talk or friendly noises. Senile persons often "play" lengthy programs of this kind, exactly repeated even though their memory is so faulty they forget they have just said the same thing moments before. And as we have noted, any downshifting tends to limit speech to repetition, probably of often-used phrases.

At the other extreme, a good many people are capable of low-repeat speech. The ability of the brain to find and select words from tens of thousands stored, to arrange them in acceptable syntactical order, and to utter them not only with clarity but with meaningful pacing and inflection, loading the words with nonverbal signals—and to do all this with little error, at a high rate of speed—must surely be counted among its most impressive achievements. How is it done?

Again we can suspect that the stored words are found by the same kind of categorizing down, and switches are thrown that put the corresponding speech motor programs into effect. But if the process were that limited, the most important or significant words would emerge first. We actually hear this happen when a person, especially a child, is under stress or very excited and trying to convey a message. The words tumble out. But ordinarily the sense of pattern, so essential to recognition of speech, inhibits the motor process long enough to rack up the words in the right order. We now know that infants do not learn to speak by imitating their elders, but individually invent and develop their own syntax—strong evidence that the sense of syntax is built into the organization of the cortical areas that handle speech.[6] It appears we store words as forms of speech. When we misspeak, saying such things as "I want to toast the newspaper" at breakfast, we are not likely to say "I want to bread the newspaper." We substitute verb for verb, noun for noun. In proster terms, they are separately stored with a regularity to gladden a grammarian's heart.[7]

If these considerations put us on the right track, it follows that we think *with* words a great deal, but very little *in* words. They are marvelously handy for marker and classifier and clue use and can be used in the natural PAC mode these ways with great ease. But thinking in verbal terms, or pushing words around, is hard work and distressingly slow. We have to do this labor when we know that what we are writing may be looked at critically—and most people find writing very trying, difficult work. The same effect occurs when an inexperienced person talks to an audience. In part downshifting ties the tongue, but usually more than that is involved. The speaker who talks naturally has little problem, but the one who tries to shift to SSM organized talk may find it cruelly exhausting and frustrating —because a deliberate effort is made *not* to use well-established programs.

In our society we have been sadly brainwashed into overrespecting SSM and greatly undervaluing PAC. The same applies to communication. The informational content of words tends to be enormously exaggerated, while the concomitant signals and clues that actually give them meaning are ignored or played down. In education and training especially, the huge error is made of stressing SSM speech and writing; the student is forced to use the most difficult and least rewarding kind of communication, under stress which adds even more obstacles. Often, in fact, the effort to practice SSM does not even involve genuine communication, but rather the student speaks or writes not to convey a message or to influence the views of another person, but merely so that the effort can be evaluated.[8]

Unless considerable observation fails me badly, those in instructional roles in our educational institutions (aside from communications specialists) rarely exhibit even a glimmer of insight into the vast difference between nonsituational and situational communication. Characteristically, teachers are baffled by the gross failure of their efforts to communicate when they attempt to use respectable SSM approaches. SSM emphasis is strong in most methods of teaching reading, with consequences all too familiar and lamentable.

And overall, as if to implement an apparent determination to do everything as wrongly as possible, the conventional school makes "stop talking!" its most frequent order, and firmly resists all real student communication. The student is imprisoned for years in an institution that discourages the constant and natural use of symbols, yet sets as its main avowed goal precisely the symbol skills it hobbles and inhibits! And to set a cherry upon the whipped cream, it quite successfuly convinces most children *not* to respect their natural ability, but to render themselves "failures" by suppressing it. The school simply carries to extreme lengths the absurdly false idea of stimulus-response. Focusing on one input, yanked out of context, it strives for an inhuman, computerlike exactitude. The isolated "right answer" is constantly sought.

But the human brain does not work that way. It does not isolate, but compares; it is built to handle comparisons—for alikeness and differences—by the billions. Our ability to recognize a word even when spoken by dozens of persons with differences in pronunciation, intonation, speed, pitch, and timbre rests on the brain's minimal reliance on any one input, and instead on the found agreement among many channels. It works as flexibly as it does precisely because it does not find isolated right answers, but functions happily by sloppy approximations—provided it can get enough approximations. This reliance on multiple near-guesses rather than one right answer is the very core of the human quality of our thinking and behavior.

To repeat, the brain is active, not passive; aggressive, not meekly waiting for stimuli. We understand speech, in essence, the same way we keep a car in lane while driving: we project an estimate of where the car will go—and of what the speaker will say; we get feedback and correct our estimate; and we repeat this cycle rapidly, over and over.[9]

We read much the same way, constantly compiling and comparing all the clues, including the size of the word and initial sound, projecting what we expect the text will say, and feeding back corrections. We have the advantage of being able to skip back to look at a past word or phrase; but actually in effect we do the same in understanding speech, by reviewing short-term memory of what was said. The skillful reader has no difficulty giving ample expression when reading aloud to text not previously seen, because the words voiced lag well behind words or patterns projected and at least partially verified by feedback. Otherwise such reading would be impossible—for example, a question mark could catch us by surprise, and we would be quite unable to build the phrase up with a rising inflection that signals a question.

We do not read as an optical-scanning computer does, focusing on each letter and recognizing it; nor even by recognizing and voicing one word at a time. Our neocortex is a pattern-recognizing instrument. Not too surprisingly, we speak, understand speech, and read in human fashion, using the various astonishing capabilities of the human brain.

Children usually learn to grasp and then use speech with quite amazing ease, considering the staggering tasks involved, because adults do not try to teach them. Unfortunately, the same is not commonly true of reading. Adults who haven't the foggiest notion of how the brain works attempt to teach, with much SSM emphasis. The result is the disaster, usually permanent in effect, that we politely call the reading problem. I submit that conventional reading instruction is the prime enemy of reading skills.

CHAPTER 18

Memory: Nowhere and Everywhere

I SHOW YOU a phonograph record. It is, we can readily agree, one example of what we have termed a program.

What is the program and how did it get there? In this case a symphony orchestra played a certain composition sometime in the past, which is now frozen in the form of bumps and wiggles in the spiral grooves. This program, then, is a memory of that performance. As such, it is *past* tense.

Now I put this record on a turntable, and the music at once is re-created, much like the original. This is happening now—*present* tense.

I turn the volume down and ask you if you can tell me what is soon to come. You know the symphony, and you hum the passage. I turn the volume up again, and in a moment we hear just what you predicted. Clearly then this program has plans or intentions—*future* tense.

This concept of a program being past, present, and future is simple enough, yet it may be confusing and even disturbing if the whole idea of program has not become familiar by frequent use in some way. In ordinary usage, memory and plan seem to be quite different concepts, in fact at opposite poles. But when we deal with programs— and the brain deals with nothing but programs, arranged in prosters —we get a sort of mental jolt at seeing tense suddenly become so slippery.

For untold centuries, memory has been regarded as a specific brain function, and it is still common to speak of improving one's memory as if it were a particular component. If we explore a large computer installation, we do find enamelled boxes containing whirling drum or disk memories; and hidden away are other memories consisting of tiny washers strung on a grid of wires. More data may be held on tape or punch cards or by several newer means.

But here computer and brain part company. If Proster Theory is on the right track and the brain is stocked with programs arranged in prosters, in turn arranged very flexibly in hierarchies, then the notion of memory as something separate makes no sense at all. *A program does not have tense, except as it is being used in one way or another as of the moment.*

If memory were a particular part of the brain, it would have some location. But while stimulating certain parts of the brain electrically can in some instances replay memories, this seems to be a switching-on function. Evidence is abundant that memory as a function does not have a specific location in the brain; nor do specific bits of memory. Enormous amounts of animal and human brains can be cut out, or destroyed by lesions or lack of blood supply, without destroying memory—as we would expect if it had location. "In the laboratory the brain seems to mock the ingenuity of the experimenter," Pribram has commented.[1] Animal brains have been sectioned, sliced, cross-hatched, laced with insulating materials, and otherwise insulated without wiping out behaviors that prove memory remains. In fact, such subjects often continue to display a high degree of skill and behave in ways that to the casual observer seem quite within the bounds of normality.

For this great riddle there is a potential answer, one that fits nicely with the concepts I have advanced. Take a square of window screening a few inches on a side and hold it in front of the screening on a window, so that the two are close. As you move the square, rotating it or changing the angle, interference patterns form, changing with the slightest movement. We see the same effect at times on television, as when in a close-up the horizontal lines of the picture interfere with a pattern in the jacket worn by an announcer.

Scientists have long used this interference pattern principle for a variety of practical purposes. With the advent of the laser and its capability of producing coherent light beams, much progress has been made in the technology called holography, which produces a physical record of what has been photographed by capturing the interference patterns of two light sources instead of the one in conventional photography. The resulting hologram is a transparent sheet with no trace of picture, only allover swirls. But putting a coherent beam through this hologram re-creates the original diffusion of light and the viewer sees the scene, not flat as on a photograph but three-dimensionally. If the viewer sees a tree is partially blocking sight of a person in the scene, he can look from another angle and see around the tree—as though he were actually on the spot![2]

If we cut a corner off a photo and lose the rest of the picture, the corner gives us no information about the whole. But the corner of a hologram will give us the entire picture, though not quite so sharply. Even a small sample of the interference pattern recorded will serve to re-create the scene.

Mathematically, the principle of interference applies without regard to the content of the patterns. That is to say any kind of information can be stored this way. Many scientists, inventors, and engineers are hot on this trail, and it seems apparent that a holographic revolution will be upon us shortly as one more in the series that have rapidly reshaped our world. As a memory device, the hologram offers enormous possibilities: billions of bits of data can be stored in a cube that can rest on a fingernail.

Pribram[3] and other investigators of the brain see in the inter-ference principle an explanation that fits many findings about the brain. Quite striking, too, is the scarcity of other possible explanations that fit the ability of the brain to operate after massive destruction. Cats, for example, could discriminate between similar optical clues after another noted experimenter, Robert Galambos, had severed up to 98 percent of the optic tract!

The mechanism of memory remains far from clear. Much evidence now suggests that long-term memory is essentially molecular, and that protein formation is involved. The role of the glia cells is part of the intricate puzzle; they compose about half the mass of the brain and their number is put at a minimum of one hundred billion. They were long thought to be merely the supporting structure for neurons, but one may well suspect that nature is far too parsimonious to squander this much material for so passive a purpose. More likely they serve several functions, of which place-holding and perhaps steering neuron extensions may be two, and assisting in the memory protein-building process another. If they have a direct memory purpose, as seems probable, their number helps make less fantastic the brain's memory capacity.

Much of the mechanism of genetic memory has been clarified by the work on deoxyribonucleic acid (DNA) and ribonucleic acid (RNA). Not only does the single cell from which a baby develops contain, in an amino acid combination code, the full "blueprints" which organize the entire individual as a unique person, but very recently it has been demonstrated that every cell carries a duplicate set. Nuclei of skin cells of adult frogs, put into frog eggs, produced adult frogs! To suppose that nature, having developed this exquisite mechanism for genetic memory (or reproductive program) purposes should also have a second, different system for the brain is to strain credulity. It seems a safe guess that mental memory will turn out to use much the same DNA/RNA procedures to record data about interference patterns pervasively throughout the brain. One such DNA molecule can hold information that in printed form would fill a good-sized library.[4]

I have emphasized that proster is a model concept, not a physical entity in a particular part of the brain. I have also stressed the role of cross-modalities, the comparison of sensory codes from different sources. It follows that hierarchies of prosters would inevitably extend pervasively. If the brain stores memory traces "where they happen," it would store them almost everywhere. For analogy, consider a large retail chain with hundreds of units that sends out to managers a memo relating to paper goods, which all of them sell. The memo would soon be widely distributed. Another memo to all stores concerns a pricing policy; it would apply to paper goods. A third memo concerns shipping claims, and also applies to paper goods. So in each store's office there would be an accumulating group of memos relevant to these products. If 99 percent of the stores were by some circumstance to lose all their information relating to paper goods, the remaining 1 percent could still supply it. In the brain, to parallel the thought very crudely, information about squirrels could be widely distributed in relation to fur, trees, nuts, climbing, backyards, and rodents. The information is thus widely distributed and heavily redundant.

Figure 14 may help us visualize this sort of distribution. At left is the common analogy for memory: a fact or bit of data which is

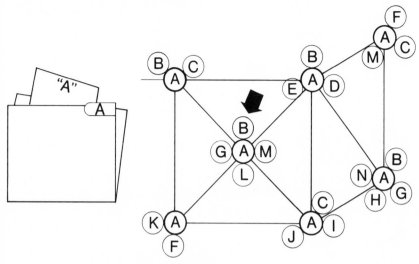

Figure 14

filed in an indexed folder. If the fact is put into the right folder (in our terms, if it is properly addressed) it can then be recovered by an inquiry to that folder (that is, if the inquiry is also properly addressed). A large file room is, of course, a capacious memory of exactly this kind.

But we must assume that the brain works quite differently, on a *network* basis as indicated, purely diagrammatically, at right. The bit of data A is stored not at one point but rather, as in our chain store analogy, at many hundreds or thousands of points. Other bits, indicated by the other letters, are also stored in various combinations at such points. Now imagine a pattern of impulses moving through the network which is "tuned" to A, as a musical note is tuned to a tuning fork. The search pattern will not only find many of the As, but can find As in combination with Bs or Cs or in certain groups. Thus a sought combination such as "ABGLM" can be found (arrow) at many locations.

The capacity and flexibility of such an arrangement is apparent even from this small network segment, with only seven junctions shown. Picture the capacity of a three-dimensional network having such junctions by the billions!

I must stress that the diagram shown merely illustrates the idea of network and not the actual structure of the brain, about which much has been learned. The overall evidence, even where there are major issues to be resolved, strongly supports the concepts of diffusion, of networks, of patterns and pattern recognition—the matching of programs we have already examined. If we study the network diagram for a moment, we can see easily how such an arrangement can link bread with butter, baker, loaf, toast; toast with toaster, breakfast; breakfast with morning, and so on through endless chains. (This is far from the S-R association of psychology a generation ago.)

Consider the file-folder idea of memory. To recall, we must have the precise label on the folder, unless we have a similarly arranged cross-index which will allow us to find it from a few other clues. A business letter in the office files, for example, may be under the name of the company, the name of the sender, or the subject matter of the letter. Such a system gives a very limited number of ways of addressing the recall. By comparison, the network system gives potentially thousands of pathways to recall.

But in either case, the addressing at the time of filing is critical. Filing the letter under the wrong heading will make it virtually irretrievable, save by luck. The danger is far less with the network; but if the strong, direct linkages are wrong, the weaker, roundabout pathways may make recall difficult. If I learn *for* a meeting or exam, addressing strongly that way, I may find the material hard to recover for other purposes.

Present knowledge suggests that we create an engram, or physical record, of *everything* that gets through the lower filters or switching centers. As we have seen, the great bulk of brain activity goes on without any need to come into the spotlight of conscious attention, which can basically accommodate only one thing at a time. An interrupted program or abortion gets full attention, as do some sensory inputs—for example pain, or some object moving in certain ways within our field of view. And we give attention to novel inputs, almost automatically, that demand a special-case program-selection decision. Engrams provide long-term memory; for practical purposes, lifetime long. Presumably, if an engram was made, no forgetting actually ensues in the sense that the trace fades out or wears out, unless physical deterioration occurs.

Under hypnosis, which facilitates recall, we may be able to recite much of a menu we inspected a week ago; and a bricklayer (as in an actual case) may be led to recall specific bricks of unusual interest laid thirty years before—verifiable by visiting the building. Elderly people approaching senility often begin to recall childhood events in great detail, and may begin to speak a language used then but presumably forgotten for perhaps seventy or more years. On returning to a neighborhood where we once lived, we may find vivid recollections flooding in unbidden, with details we could not have provided a day before. Similarly, psychiatric therapy may bring back even very early childhood events, recaptured all too powerfully.

Very short-term memory does not seem to be engrammed at all. There is a considerable body of research that shows putting the record in permanent form takes appreciable time, counted in minutes, at least—a fact that fits the protein synthesis hypothesis. Rather, as Hebb long ago suggested, such brief memory may exist in the form of reverbatory circuits, impulses going around and around a complex loop.

If we probe back into our origins by the need technique, it seems apparent that any creature that has a nervous system and that moves must be able to tell whether *it* is moving in relation to its surroundings: is it swimming toward a shadow, or is the shadow approaching? The answer is essential to interpret sensory input. The creature must then be aware of what it is doing or has just done; and it is not easy to see much distinction between such an awareness and "consciousness." At a higher level, an animal such as a field mouse, subject to sudden attack, must know what refuges it has just passed. Current memory, covering the last few minutes, appears essential to survival, but very quickly, usually, the information becomes of no value.

We see then the need for a filter, or a switching center that will allow the transient memory to terminate and be replaced with more recent input—unless the content is recognized (that is, matches an existing program) and evaluated, in the light of experience, (by prosters for this purpose) as having importance. In that event, it is switched into circuits that will permit engramming or registration. Much progress has been made in identifying these switching areas and tracing the flow of input. Since they are predominantly in the older brains, they do not "trust" the neocortex under strong stress. As noted, our recollection of stressful happenings tends to be crude, sadly lacking in detail. From this downshifting, too, comes the "unreasoning" fears many people have, deriving from incidents perhaps going back to early childhood. There may be fear of boating or swimming, of fire, of certain animals, foods, tools, materials—quite reptilian memories that discriminate poorly and can be very hard to overcome. The older the brain, the cruder the memory, the broader the program of avoidance.

Short-term memory can be so brief that by the time we have

finished dialing a phone number we cannot recall it. Or, in a quite low-pressure social circumstance, we are introduced to two friends of a friend, and two minutes later cannot recall the name of either. On the other hand, we seem to be able to recall many trivial events or details of the day. It seems likely that we have some medium-term kind of function, perhaps based on molecules that do forget by a process of chemical decay similar to wiping clean a bit of magnetic tape so it can be used again. The evidence in this area is much less well developed. We do seem to be able to keep mental notes in some fashion. I can resolve to "call George this week," and carry out the program perhaps three days hence; or determine that I must visit a museum when I get a chance, and do so some weeks later.

A strikingly common, if unscientific, observation of medium-term memory relates to conscious, vigorous, SSM learning. If a person gathers some facts prior to a meeting, not because they interest him but because he feels they might be asked for, he is likely to find that after the meeting they have vanished with astonishing completeness. The phenomenon is highly noticeable in schooling. Students at all levels cram or are crammed for tests; give a good many remembered answers; but soon after, to the everlasting dismay of teachers, behave almost as if they had never heard of the material. The final examination, on which much of the grade awarded often rests, usually turns out to be final indeed. Rarely do schools, even though their psychologists define learning as a lasting change, check back three or six months later to see how much was retained. Such evidence as we have, from a variety of studies, suggests that in those areas where the students would not be too likely to have much input from outside of school, retention proves startlingly low. After ten years of studying mathematics, for example, high school seniors typically have only a feeble grasp of elementary arithmetic.

A considerable and growing body of experimental evidence indicates that the mechanisms of memory present unexpected puzzles. Laboratory animals appear to remember training for a number of minutes, then lose memory sharply for a few hours, only to regain it many hours later and retain it for days. This "Kamin effect," as it is called, and some remarkable investigations in which RNA brain extracts from trained animals had bizarre effects on recipients (often producing results opposite from what logic would dictate), strongly suggest that in the consolidating of memory there are, as universally throughout the body, forces pulling in opposite directions.[5] We can speculate that short-term memory gets a head start, then some "anti" factor begins to have a wipe-out effect, and the resulting combat can end either with little trace left, or with long-term engrams firmly established.

In any case, the old simplistic notions of a "curve of forgetting" and "extinction" can no longer be taken seriously.

The reader who boggled at Proster Theory's distinction between natural, efficient PAC and clumsy SSM modes may be even more astonished when we consider the difference as it affects memory. When subjects are asked to remember a sequence of digits or letters that make no sense, or are given similar tasks, they can recall only a small number for a very brief period; much forgetting begins in a few seconds. Pure symbols are exceedingly difficult to retain. But other experiments show that if subjects are shown 2,500 pictures at the rate of one every ten seconds, in sessions over days, and then shown many pairs of pictures, one new and one previously shown, they can identify the one seen before with very high accuracy, days and weeks and months later![6] Memory for pictures seems to be almost limitless and highly durable. Pictures, of course, are pure PAC.

Similarly, we may note that young children can often repeat the words of a television commercial to perfection—until they learn to read. Once symbols take the place of patterns, the PAC ability becomes seriously hampered.

Our remarkable inability to remember isolated symbols appears to confirm the concept of memory as the past-tense aspect of programs. We remember long-term by establishing programs, and no program, or no program that can be located by search, means no memory. And inherent in the nature of programs is the concept of chains: each element is linked; none stands isolated.

But if we examine the idea of symbol more than casually, we see that we apply that word over a continuum of fixed meaning. Our flag, for instance, is a symbol of our country; a most specific meaning. But a white flag, in the proper setting, symbolizes surrender or truce or "let's talk," which are much less specific meanings. When we proceed down the continuum and come to "x" or "8" we deal with pure symbols. It takes a good deal of time to teach a child or an illiterate that this kind of symbol *doesn't* mean anything specific— that 8 may mean 8 peas or 8 elephants or an abstract eightness. The usefulness of pure symbols lies in this attribute. I can use 8x now and 8x an hour from now to mean entirely different things. If the symbols held meaning, as does our flag, they would be most difficult to manipulate—and that is what pure symbols are for.

The more we go toward SSM thinking, the more we are dealing with pure symbols that shed meaning as some silicone-treated surface sheds water. We can retain symbols, such as a formula or telephone number, only by embedding them in nonsymbolic programs. To aid memory, when we are told a number we usually write it down; or if we read it, we repeat it aloud, thus using cross-modal programs to help recall. Mnemonic devices such as "thirty days hath September . . . ," or "FACE" and "every good boy deserves favor" for the notes of the treble clef, use this principle of embedding. Since words are organized on the left side of the cortex and music on the right side (in most people's brains), use of a tune is highly cross-modal, and a strong pattern as well—as the persistence of television jingles and the songs of years ago readily proves.

On a larger scale, we can gain new insight into the learning-by-doing concept, so often associated with John Dewey, but also embraced intuitively by a long list of outstanding educators over many centuries. Doing means embedding, making use of cross-modalities, and ideally, the discovery and employment of patterns. And out of the process comes appropriate, broad addressing, a multitude of pathways that permit the categorizing-down search process to locate the pertinent stored programs richly and rapidly. The more intricately *textured* learning becomes, the more the access channels multiply.

Learning for the purpose of answering examination questions usually involves only very limited responses to specific questions, or arbitrary manipulations of symbols. Educators have long been aware that evaluation tends to focus on what is easy and convenient to evaluate, not what is most meaningful. Equally, they know that instruction tends to be shaped by the anticipated evaluation; the teacher tries to prepare the student to pass the exam or show up well on the achievement test, which is merely another, convenient form of exam. Business and industrial training, though often poorly planned and executed, at least more commonly aims at useful learning. But it is precisely the failure to embed and create a texture that creates the boredom and unhappiness of the assembly-line worker or clerk or soldier, and the alienation of the young citizen who cannot fit observations of society into a texture of which he or she seems a part. While they may learn by doing, they fail to learn *what* they are doing.

Engramming, since it involves a molecular change, requires energy, just as it takes energy to put molecules into a certain arrangement on a magnetic tape for sound reproduction. This suggests a general mechanism that appears to provide a neat reluctance on the part of the brain to accept unnecessary engrams. We may suspect that inputs that get through the initial filtering do not become permanently engrammed unless they provide the minimum energy required, though it need not be supplied all at once.

Common experience tells us that engramming can occur by a sudden, important incident; although if strong threat was involved, there may have been downshifting that eliminated much detail. Presumably such events provided a surge of energy ample to engram at one exposure.

Rote learning falls at the other extreme. Repeated input, though inconsequential and unexciting, has its cumulative effect. We come to know a symphony, for example, by repeated hearings; or we can clearly recall the details of a route we often walked long before, or a building we went to daily. The energy input on each exposure was low, but cumulative.

In between, we seem to engram by fewer repeats of moderate intensity. For example, if we have to visit a doctor a number of times for treatment, we may establish a vivid memory of him and his office and the procedures.

While the present state of knowledge does not permit more than speculation on the point, this energy test has an appealing simplicity, and seems to fit neatly with the evolutionary need approach. Possibly, too, it throws light on a group of baffling findings long known to "reinforcement" psychologists: that administering electrical shocks —presumably punishment—when an animal made the right response in a learning test actually appeared to help it learn; and to make matters worse, shocks for either right or wrong answers also seemed to contribute. This held true even in experiments using human learners.[7] If we view the punishment as additional energy input, the awkward findings at last make sense.

Here too multiple addressing and access play a part. Whether the energy comes along a main avenue of interproster connections or around "back roads" would matter little; only the total delivered to one point would matter. For analogy, consider a broad campus lawn over which students walk to various surrounding buildings. The grass will become most worn down where paths intersect—where energy accumulates. Those paths that get used by many students will tend to become wider, for the same reason.

But in any discussion of memory we must bear in mind the fundamental nature of the brain's apparatus: its reliance on clueing, on comparative and differential analysis, on contexts and patterns, and not on isolated hard bits of data. Most of what we remember is skimpy and fuzzy, as the disagreements of several participants in an event some years later will attest. We tend to recall in ways that, by remarkable coincidence, suit our current purpose or convenience. As some famous memory-expert cases show, too good a memory can be painful, and a liability. To have the flexibility to deal with the present—the greatest of human qualities—an imperfect recollection is a requisite. Too often we encounter people whose memory, so to speak, has hardened, and who exhibit a rigidity of thought and behavior and resistance to modifying programs or acquiring new ones even when the need seems pressing. "They live in the past," we say— a misuse of memory.

Memory, to summarize, is the past-tense aspect of program. What we term recall is simply a shift of tense to the present. Programs do not exist, within our theory, in isolation, but only in prosters, infinitely linked with other prosters in hierarchies. Memory, then, is equally distributed and pervades the brain—the more so as multiple modalities are involved, since touch, sight, hearing, smell, and so on have different organizing areas in the brain.

Addressing, as we have seen, is crucial to ability to use stored programs in the present: the address when the memory is engrammed and the address when recall is sought must at least roughly match. And the more the program is embedded, and richly linked with other prosters, the broader and more varied the address channels can be.

Engramming probably depends on the use of a critical minimum amount of energy, either on one occasion or accumulated.

With these concepts, we can approach learning with some practical idea of how to bring it about.

CHAPTER 19

The Very Human Image Within

Consider me for a moment as twentieth-century man, as I make plans for the coming day. I set my clock to assure my waking in good time. After dressing and eating and walking the dog, I will have an hour to gather and arrange some material, and make two phone calls. Then I will head for New York and some business over lunch with an old friend. Following that, a stop to pick up some photos, and another stop at the library to check a reference. If I get back in time, I will finish an article in progress. After dinner, there is a concert at 8:30, and if certain friends are met, a short visit with them at a restaurant nearby. Then home, some reading, and to bed.

Now shift the scene to a hunting band, 15,000 years ago. Game has been scarce. An expedition has been planned to start at dawn the next morning. Weapons and the few supplies to be carried have been checked and made ready. The party will head north, over the ridge; if no game is found it will go to a long valley beyond that; and if necessary it will hunt to the south. If meat is obtained fairly close it will be brought back, but if a lot of game is come upon, a messenger will be sent back to bring the whole clan to the new location. If luck is bad, the hunters will return by the end of the third day.

Planning of this kind, for a day, a week, a month, even a year or several years, clearly falls within the powers of man today, and we have no reason to suppose the hunting band was any less competent. If they had no wristwatches, they managed nicely by glancing at the sun. Probably they cared less about small units of time, which argues that they lived better in this respect, not worse.

How are we able to formulate, retain, adjust, and execute such plans? We have seen that the future tense of program is plan, but these are programs of programs, capable of branching or substitution to meet contingencies.

We know that the brain has large "silent areas," as W. Grey Walter calls them. When these are stimulated by electric probe no motor or sensory effect results, as would be the case in other regions. The patient feels nothing, notices nothing, and activity is not affected. That the stimulation is "felt" by the brain is proved by vigorous changes in brain wave patterns as seen by the electroencephalograph. Such areas are located all over the brain, but most massively in the frontal lobes, behind the forehead, where we know sensory inputs of all modes are routed.

The history of Phineas Gage, the victim of the tamping rod, together with evidence from a great many brain operations (now seldom performed) in which frontal tissue was either removed or severed so as to disconnect segments from the rest of the brain, gives a good general idea of the function of this large portion of the cortex. When both frontal lobes are inoperative, the patient becomes, in Dr. Walter's words, "torpid, inert, unimaginative, and irresponsible."[1] In common language, he stops worrying. Such patients can carry on many activities and even seem quite pleasant, relaxed companions. But the sense of planning, drive, and concern for the future that is eminently human simply disappears. Mr. Gage, the overzealous foreman, lost enough of his frontal lobes to become undependable, an aimless drifter.

On the level of broad generalizations, supported by a mass of observations, we can say with some confidence that this "frontal characteristic" seems to feed and grow stronger on certain types of experience. To review even the main experimental evidence here would be too great a task; but it strongly suggests that frontal-lobe development, along with that of all the silent organizing areas, can be greatly arrested or distorted if the child does not get what is needed during the early years.

These needs fall rather easily under three headings. The first appears to be, in essence, *input*: the child requires a huge, varied, and preferably heavily cross-modal mass of sensory experiences. Just what it sees, hears, feels, and so on apparently does not matter too much; quantity and variety count more than what adults might consider quality. But it is a safe guess that *reality* matters, and that the reality content of the overall input should be high. It is good for a child to hear various sounds, including the sound of a bell; but it is better for him to see the bell shaken to produce the sound, or to handle it himself. Reality assures the cross-modality that facilitates learning. The adult can listen to an orchestra via radio and mentally picture the players and instruments that produced the sound, but the infant only hears sound. Someone playing a guitar in its presence provides quite a different set of inputs. The brain, as we have seen, is a comparative and differential analysis device, and it cannot compare or note differences when given a single input.

The dominance of brain and input is revealed by two familiar pieces of evidence. Hopi Indians commonly raised children on cradle-boards, slung on the mothers' backs, which greatly limited the infants' movements during most of their waking day. What effect would this have on their learning to walk? One might think that it would greatly delay the achievement; but studies showed nothing of the kind occurred. The cradled children walked at the same age range as children not cradled.[2] But we should note that the cradle-board (like some of the new devices parents widely use) permitted the babies to be exposed to a great variety of real inputs as the women went about their daily business. The infants were in an ideal posture to see, hear, smell, feel, and sense motion and changes in position.

In contrast, studies of children in an orphanage in Teheran, who were given little attention or activity, showed shocking retardation. At two years of age more than half could still not sit up alone, and at four 85 percent still could not walk—at two to four times the usual age.[3] Many animal (including primate) experiments confirm the deadly effect of deprivation of sensory experience during the early period of development. I am not speaking here of children being taught or getting selected input, but of obtaining a great variety of commonplace, largely real, random input. Any teaching effort would seem likely to be at least ineffective and at worst very hazardous. It is one thing to give an infant rich exposure, quite a different thing to try to control that exposure when we have far too little knowledge of just how the development proceeds, and when we do know that the needs of each child differ over an enormous range.

The second cluster of needs can be listed under *security*, although with some reservations about that term. The security must be from the infant's point of view, not the adult's. The child explores and becomes familiar with the strange, confusing world it has been born into by moving out from a base, which initially is normally the mother's cherishing and protective presence. Much of the sense of security derives, it seems plain, from the child's knowledge that the base can be returned to at any time. As a child matures, it essays expeditions further and further from base; and it also widens the concept of base, from the personal presence and touch of the mother to family, and home, and familiar ground. Eventually security can become an inner confidence.

On this score there is substantial evidence that the child (or young animal) that encounters moderately traumatic experiences early becomes better able to cope with difficulties later. It is hardly news that overprotection of youngsters can take a toll, but it is useful to know that some degree of "suffering," if not overwhelming, does indeed seem to build what used to be called character. Some of the character-building enthusiasts should note, however, that such traumatic events need only be few and occasional. One may doubt that a daily cold shower, or equivalent, does much for the frontal lobes.

The third group of needs may be labeled *social*. One of the few built-in schemata (the beginnings of programs that are present at birth) is response to a face, or anything like a face.[4] We are social animals. People are of enormous importance to us, which is why we so frequently see interpersonal conflicts. To a large degree people provide real inputs for an infant, since it will give attention to a person approaching rather than to almost anything else. Even while only days old, a baby picks up signals of some subtlety from those who hold it or touch it, and before long from tone of voice or rapidity of movement of hand, arm, or other part of the older person's body. Long prior to much command of speech, the child can normally send and receive nonverbal signals with ease and accuracy. It has become well aware of different levels and kinds of relationships with different people, which is to say it has developed considerable social skill.

We tend to take for granted this crucially important learning and development, to the point of being mystified when confronted with children whose needs have not been met, and who become the victims of such labels as retarded, disturbed, learning disabled, hyperactive, withdrawn, minimally brain damaged, and others that are all too easily pasted on a child. Until quite recently the notion persisted

—and still does, in sometimes astonishing places—that the child matures by some inner time clock and so what happens before the clock sounds its signal is of no importance. As the Teheran orphans so pathetically dramatize, the maturing occurs only if the needs have been met. The idea, still common among those who deal with young children, of "wait for the maturity and then teach" fails to recognize that it is not teaching that matters (except as it can do harm) during the early building of the amazing frontal apparatus, but the needs I have named: abundant sensory input, especially cross-modal and real; a sense of security or base; and the interplay with various people that becomes the raw material of social skills. Basically, these are deep-seated, old-brain needs.

As we can see in Figure 15, a very large portion of the new brain consists of what are called, perhaps for lack of any better name, association or organizing areas—silent in Walter's sense.[5] These are not the only organizing parts of the brain, which filters and selects and organizes at every level and in many general locations; but these cortical areas are by all evidence *not* concerned with the initial reception of sensory input or with the sending of orders to the muscles— the old telephone plug-board concept—but rather with far broader interpretation and evaluation. They deal with the question, "What does this input mean in the light of my experience and what should I do about it?" The process of seeing, for example, involves first the detection of bits and pieces of visual information, such as edges at various rotations from the vertical. These fragments must then be assembled to make sense of what the eyes have viewed. The occipital lobes, at the very back of the skull, have this function.

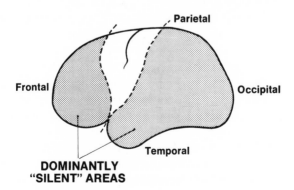

Figure 15

We can feel fairly certain that the question asked by the frontal lobes is something like, "How does this current situation fit with my long-term concept of myself and my world?" If the fit is tolerably good, sense of security is bolstered. If the fit is marginal (and that is the precise word), accommodations must be made, by revising aspects of the previous concept, or by reinterpreting the new situation with some change, or both. If instead there is a gross misfit, other means of coping must be employed. The simplest, and the most usual, is to ignore or reject. If we have no established recognition proster for the new input, we of course cannot perceive it; like the words of a foreign language, it lacks meaning. Ignoring raises no problem. But if there is enough recognition along various channels to prevent this easy avoidance, recourse may be to filter the unwanted, awkward information out, or suppress it. This kind of higher-level filtering, we can strongly suspect, reflects an important function of the frontal apparatus.

This ability not to see what we don't want to see is a common theme of humor, as illustrated by the quip, "I read that smoking was bad for my health, so I gave up reading," or the sign that hangs in offices, "My mind is made up—kindly do not bother me with the facts." But all too often it has tragic implications: the amateur singer who loves to perform and cannot hear his or her off-pitch tones or strained high notes, the father who blinds himself to his son's inability or disinclination to follow in his footsteps, the manager who utterly fails to recognize the consequences of his actions, or the person in any of a thousand settings who cannot realize and admit that old, long relied-on ways have become outmoded. Arthur Miller's *Death of a Salesman* dramatizes the pain and shattering effect of being forced to open the filter and let the rejected information in.

Any such forced revision of one's self-image, even if positive, can be painful and destructive. Many a psychiatrist treats successes, especially those who rose rapidly; and the achievement of retirement notoriously may be followed by depression and illness. If Proster Theory is on the right track, the explanation goes beyond the obvious one of being deflated by failure, worried about maintaining success, or bored by inactivity. We enter here the area that has been explored by some psychologists as "cognitive dissonance."[6]

I have advanced the concept of programs being aborted in the process of execution and the consequent alarm and immediate shift of attention to the aborted program. If I am reading a book while munching on a meat sandwich, I pay utterly no attention to how I chew; but if my teeth close on a bit of bone, the abortion will instantly bring attention. We could say that dissonance exists between the pattern of normal chewing and the pattern occasioned by the hard particle. In the same vein, I have stated that the matching of input with recognition prosters need not be exact. Some tolerance is allowed; accuracy comes from comparing many clues. But where there is a good, firm match in part of the pattern recognition, and in other parts a failure to match, we again have an abortion with acute dissonance. I like to call this the Santa Claus effect, recalling the dismay of a neighbor who dressed in that costume, intending to please his young children. The moment he spoke they became terrified and badly upset—the familiar voice and nonverbal signals and the strange beard and clothes created unbearable dissonance, or in our present terminology a gross recognition abortion.

Man's frontal lobes, we have much reason to believe, serve as a sort of stabilizer. Here must develop the highly complex evaluation prosters which recognize intricate, slow, long-term programs. When the boss chews out the employee at close range, the old brain signals attack; the middle brain signals anger; but the frontal lobes refuse to be stampeded and consider the paycheck, the cost of groceries, the payments on the car, and the prospect of eventual promotion to a desired job. Usually, the boss escapes damage. We could not be the social beings we are, or tolerate the frustrating world civilization keeps us in, without some such control in the brain.

The higher up we go in the phylogenic scale, the more complex is the environment lived in, and the longer the learning period provided. The human offspring is born into a tremendously intricate world, with a bare minimum of built-in programs and the need to construct a staggeringly large number to make sense of the inputs that flood in. We have to look at learning periods, the plastic stages, as tolerant of a great deal of dissonance. We can say that the youngster has a license to be ignorant. "I don't know" can be an acceptable answer to many questions, as well as "I have not had that experience" expressed in some form; children in school will chorus "we haven't *had* that!" as an unarguable reason for not knowing. Gradually, what can be termed a *tolerable level of ignorance* is pushed down in one area after another, and in these, displaying ignorance becomes embarrassing.

At the same time, on a parallel line of development, self-image becomes more precise and hardens as the early plasticity is slowly lost. We see this plainly enough through simple observation, particularly in rearing our own children. The process continues in our society into early adulthood; we speak of young men and women "finding themselves," or "discovering who they are."

Such language is vague, and even suspect. But in brain terms, we can put forward a principle that in one sense sums up much of the discussion of brain functions we have considered so far: the concept of *regeneration*. MacLean's analogy of the television receiver will serve well. In a studio, a television camera scans a scene, transduces it to a coded pattern of impulses which are broadcast and then to a degree regenerated to form a picture on our home TV screen. The picture formed by a good set seems clear and realistic, but of course it is very crude compared to the original, and distorted in various ways. We have no trouble recognizing this regeneration even if it distorts the original scene into tones of gray, or, on a color set, into hues obviously not true to the original. If the signal received is weak and the receiver of poor quality, the regenerated picture may deteriorate to vague shapes, and, at worst, to meaningless confusion.

The brain transduces the original scene, our individual environment, to patterns of impulses, and these must then be regenerated into a "picture" to have meaning. The picture will be of relatively poor quality and distorted by the mechanism—we can see only within a limited range of light wavelengths, not including ultraviolet or infrared, and hear only certain sounds, not too low or high in pitch. Just as a good television picture seems to us marvelously clear, though it is actually crude and distorted, so our internal regeneration often seems entirely adequate. If it permits us to jump a stream or thread a needle, it appears to serve our purposes. Figure 16 suggests these ideas in very simplified form.

Coded patterns are our sole means of experiencing the environment: all knowledge of it must come through this process. Just as we can turn knobs on the television receiver and bias the brightness or contrast or colors, or turn the tone control and bias the sound toward base or treble, so we constantly bias the sensory apparatus to adjust the picture inside the brain. Why do we bias? For precisely the same reason that we fiddle with the television knobs: to get what we individually think is a clearer or more pleasing regeneration.

"Learning" implies obtaining a regeneration of the world we individually live in that serves our purposes, that permits some understanding, that enables us to see how we fit in, and above all that lets us feel that we can have some confidence of survival and well-being

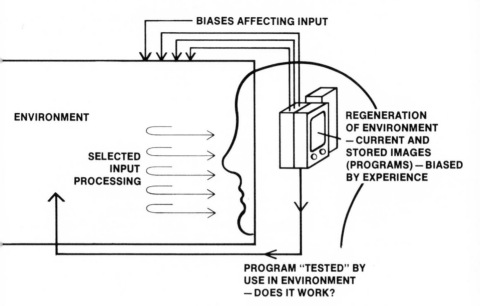

Figure 16

The rectangle represents the individual's environment. From this, certain inputs are selected for processing while others are ignored. Even those selected are modified by current brain biases, as indicated at top of diagram. Within the brain, the admitted inputs serve to regenerate a "picture" of the environment, which is further biased in the light of stored experience and expectations. The program then chosen as appropriate is put into effect and (bottom of diagram) tested by use in the environment. If the program works reasonably well, the individual feels confidence in the inner images that led to its choice. If it aborts, the individual feels threat and must either try other programs from the store available or in some way withdraw.

because the environment will, to a satisfactory degree, not spring too many surprises on us. As humans, with a far more sophisticated cortex than any other animal, we can make use of programs that total huge numbers, can be very subtle and very long, and make interconnections beyond count. Programs by nature are past, present, and future; the more elaborate the program inventory, the more a creature can live in past and future as well as present.

But utterly essential to this whole design is the trustworthiness of the regenerated image. It must serve. When it fails, when through poor input or overbiasing the internal image produces dissonance beyond normal tolerance, or simply does not deliver adequate information, the result is abortion on a scale that produces acute distress. Massive failure—as when one is forced to revise an established self-image—or continuous, frequent failure, may well have a shattering effect. This is readily demonstrable in the laboratory with animals, which can quite quickly be rendered neurotic, depressed, anxious, and poorly able to function by forcing conflicting inputs upon them, or by requiring decisions based on inadequate information (the chronic problem of the executive, who may also feel the strain!).

The confident person, the one in good mental health, the one who feels sure of being able to learn something new or to cope with complex problems, is by this view simply the one with a high degree of trust in inner images, based on the experience that executed programs seem to work—they only occasionally abort in practice. Lack of trust produces hesitancy, timidity, anxiety, depression. Abraham Maslow's "self-actuating" individual, and the great bulk of those who prove high achievers over a period of time, characteristically display enormous assurance within their own fields. At the other extreme we find the "minimally brain-damaged" child or the one with "learning disabilities." Both terms are misleading labels at times applied to individuals given so many Santa Claus inputs in early childhood that their trust in inner images becomes very low.[7]

While the frontal lobes retain much of their mystery, we can be reasonably sure that here is where the evaluation prosters and long-term programs that determine overall nature, and what we call personality, are built, modified, and established, especially during the period from about ages four to seven through about ages seventeen to twenty-two.[8]

When we view behavior in program and proster terms, with adequate respect for the unique human frontal lobes' functions, the traditional rat-in-a-box "reward and punishment" and "reinforcement" concepts that serve as cornerstones of behaviorist psychologies become absurdly simplistic. They have embarrassing gaps even with rats; applied to humans they have almost no value. They *sound* beautifully logical, and we have all been brought up with these ideas, usually presented as unquestioned; but when we examine them with rigor they collapse.

First, we cannot be thought of as free agents who can do whatever may be needed to obtain a reward. At any given time a particular person can use only those programs that have already been established. The most that can be done is to select from a proster the program that is perceived as most appropriate—it may or may not prove sufficiently suitable. Even then, the addressing to reach that proster depends on the total combination of biases applying *as of the moment*—and these include past experience (right back to earliest infancy) as well as aspirations for the future, the individual's percept of the circumstances, self-concept, current role and programs in progress, and ambient factors. All of these are interactive. To apply rat-think to the human brain, six hundred times as large and millions of times more intricate, virtually guarantees wrong answers.

Second, while the rat can press a bar and release a food pellet accidentally at first, and by a simple program thereafter, human programs almost always are long and complicated, involving dozens to hundreds or thousands of steps. The outcome, or result, or "reward" cannot often be related to simple, single acts or decisions. To drive a few miles to a friend's house, for example, I may have to make a hundred correct decisions at intersections, in sequence. Any wrong choice may abort my program (but may not, if I reach the same street at a different point); or I could make several mistakes and not know which put me off my course. The same holds true in making a business agreement, cooking a dinner, balancing a check-book, place-kicking a football, growing a lawn, tuning a car's engine, writing an essay, bringing a boat into dock, or persuading a shop-keeper to accept a check: the reward, if attained, usually throws little light on which elements of the long program worked for the outcome, or against it, or had no effect. In addition, any number of factors not in the program can affect the outcome. The business deal succeeds because of a totally unforeseen outbreak of war in another country; the dinner is spoiled by the late arrival of guests, delayed by a jammed drawbridge; the shopkeeper refuses to cash a check because he was cheated by a customer the day before.

Unlike the rat, we do not have to rely heavily on trial and error to learn. A road map will contribute greatly to making the right decisions at intersections. I can take a book out of the library on lawn growing, or enroll in a course on boat handling. (Unfortunately, such aids can also lessen success: the map or book could be out of date, or the course instructor poorly qualified.)

Further, the program itself, in human affairs, may have great importance. We carry on a hierarchy of simultaneous programs, from advancing a career to sharpening a pencil. We can, and often do, engage in conflicting programs, vacillating between goals: enjoy food, lose weight. A badly served, overpriced meal in a restaurant may outrage us more than reward us, although our hunger was relieved.

Sharply different programs may produce similar results: a skilled painter may do a room in four hours, against the sixteen a beginner might take. A machine operator who turns out virtually perfect work, but too slowly, may be discharged as too expensive to retain. You may choose to walk twice as far on an errand in order to pass a park with shrubs in bloom. Skill, grace, physical effort, esthetics are only a few of the factors that may make a program rewarding in itself. The notion of "a" reward, the equivalent of the rat's food pellet, ignores the many levels of program activity in humans, and the importance of the quality of the programs themselves.

Third, even what seem clearly rewards or punishments in the conventional sense often prove on examination to involve the same sort of complexities and ambiguities. In a sales contest, the winner is awarded a trip to Bermuda for himself and his wife. The wife wants to go, but the man fears flying—and the "reward" results in exposing his dread, and a destructive quarrel with his spouse. Millions of alcohol users suffer agonizing hangovers, automobile accidents, even arrest, loss of employment, family crises, public disgrace—yet keep on drinking. One wonders how they could be punished more, but the punishment doesn't seem to work. Consider the child learning to walk, who suffers bump after bump in falls, yet keeps trying; or the young aspiring actor who gets turned down and rebuffed again and again, yet perseveres for years on end; or the bettor who consistently loses at the racetrack yet more and more poses as an expert.[9]

The doctrine of reinforcement and the widespread belief in the efficacy of reward and punishment are among the most sacred of cows, but they give no milk. In ordinary human affairs, they offer virtually no utility. Even if they had basic validity, which seems most doubtful, human complexities would make them inapplicable.

In contrast, the concept of programs, prosters, and biases, deriving from the nature of the human brain, does give useful insights and permits applications. We can examine even complex programs in detail, or deliberately learn new ones to add to prosters. Once aware of the role of biases, we can effect planned changes that open the way to learn new ideas and behaviors.

By no means do all psychologists retain pristine faith in reinforcement. Increasingly it is viewed as at best a suspect principle.[10]

CHAPTER 20

The Bones of Proster Theory

A THEORY should result in laws. Law in this use has no implication of permanence or infallibility. On the contrary, the initial use of the law or laws deriving from a theory is to provide a concise statement of what is to be *tested*. It may be possible to devise experiments that either sustain or damage the law; and showing it to be false or faulty can be easier and faster than showing it to be true, for true is at best tentative. If direct experimentation proves difficult, the value of a law can be indirectly tested by acting as if it were true and applying it in various complex circumstances. If favorable results seem to be associated with application, at least a suspicion arises that the law may have validity.

But even without any clear outcomes that support or damage a law, it can have practical usefulness if it provides a frame of reference, a new way of looking at what we have often looked at. If I say: "Popular stringed instruments always have eight strings or some multiple of four," and you check this, you may well end with more knowledge, and even understanding, of stringed instruments than you might have had before you considered this proposition, whether or not it proves true.

In this chapter I will try to extract some laws from the broad discussion of Proster Theory that has gone before. They will have some usefulness as we turn to implications and applications in the section that follows.

1. Unity: the brain has only one basic organizational form—programs, in prosters, in hierarchies.

If this is correct, we at one stroke enormously simplify the riddle the brain presents. There should be no observable function of the brain that cannot be accounted for in this way. Admittedly, we have not considered in any depth how seeing, hearing, or speech is organized: these are beyond the scope of this book. Yet so far as I have pursued these questions elsewhere, I have found no evidence that additional processes must be presumed. On the side of unity is the stubborn preference of nature for one method, modified or elaborated, rather than several. Since all brain function evolved from the same primitive nervous tissue, unity is highly probable. The notion that the brain has a hodgepodge of different operations derives from the century of effort by great numbers of psychologists to investigate parts rather than the whole.

2. Availability: since the brain functions by programs, it can function only to the extent that programs, as of the moment, have been established.

This means that one can do only what one has previously learned to do, which seems almost too obvious to be worth setting down. But if we observe people in action, we can constantly see examples of an employer becoming angry with a worker, or a teacher annoyed by a child, precisely because they failed to do something they could not possibly do, since they lacked a program. Even so, it should be easier to recognize the absence of an externally visible program than an internal recognition program. Unaccustomed to viewing human behavior in program terms, we tend to think that everyone sees and hears as we do. They don't and they can't, of course, unless they have previously established the necessary recognition programs.

3. Foundation: all programs must be built upon existing programs.

The reason why this must be true (within Proster Theory) may be difficult to grasp at once. But it is simply a way of saying that something cannot be made from nothing. One needs letters to form a word and words to form a sentence. An input cannot be recognized or otherwise used unless there preexists in the brain some program to refer it to. Consider again the person who gains sight after years of blindness; the eyes work in the sense that light strikes the retina and impulses go to the occipital lobes, but the input is meaningless. Input can be used only insofar as it matches or approximately relates to programs already present.[1]

It follows that a child must be born with some programs already existing; we can use the accepted term "schemata" for these built-in and rather vague programs. Their presence has been well documented experimentally. The snowball effect may help to explain differences in the way children learn, and particularly the rate: very slight differences in the quality of schemata at birth would have profound influence if all learning must be built on previous learning. Again, observation suggests that we are on the right track.

The precise methods by which programs, and then prosters, are built need not be discussed here. We can note that we are speaking of the building of networks, and that we know the cortex typically is arranged three-dimensionally, with neurons often in stacks and rows and layers. We also can see that the original need for more "thinking" arose from cross-modal inputs, from handling or adjusting or reconciling two or more simultaneous inputs from different sources. This is fundamentally why there must be networks rather than localized structures. For our present purposes, we can visualize these main means by which programs elaborate and prosters and hierarchies form:

a) The program lengthens as segments are chained.
b) The program thickens—grows sideways as minor variations are accreted, perhaps eventually splitting to form the roughly parallel or alternative choices characteristic of a proster.
c) The program branches, the way a road forks.

One way to picture this process, very roughly, is to imagine a troop of army signalmen stringing wires in a forest, some high in the tree-tops, others low or on the ground, with vertical connections as required, the object being to connect scattered units and observers. If we now visualize other, adjacent troops doing the same thing, we can see that before long the various systems will begin to intertwine and ultimately connect, and increasingly establish alternative ways of sending a message from point A to point B. This is the analog of programs elaborating to build prosters, richly interconnected.

We can also see that when two of these signal systems are hooked together, there occurs a sudden and large jump in capacity. Characteristically, each of these systems grew and elaborated by adding contiguously—by adding on a few more yards of line in some direction, with one end attached to what had already been put up. This is a slow process, in contrast to the jump that occurs when two or more systems thus painfully built are joined. Few observers of learning have failed to note that learning, motor skills, problem-solving, and creative thinking (to use the conventional terms) evidence this behavior: slow, laborious accretions often showing a plateau on a progress curve, followed by a virtually instantaneous rise to a new level. The youngster struggling to ride a bicycle suddenly gets the hang of it and can balance; the inventor suddenly becomes aware of a new avenue of investigation or a solution; the novelist sees suddenly how a development can be handled.

The key word here is connection, and it gives us another law.

4. Connection: sudden increases in mental capacity occur when links are established between two or more proster networks not previously connected.

We can suspect two main factors operate to produce these new, major connections. One is fresh input, the other the process of search, especially when it is deliberately employed in a favorable setting. Both together probably have best effect.

In the neurophysiological aspects of my exploration of the brain, I have largely ignored one puzzling fact: neurons typically are given to discharging or firing quite spontaneously, without apparent rhyme or reason. Erratically, they just go off.[2] Why this should be, and what the function is, remains far from answered. Proster Theory suggests a rather obvious speculation—that the random firing serves to prevent the brain from "getting into ruts." In any case, this problem calls for some attention. Obviously, a great deal that we do from day to day reflects what are commonly called habits. It is easy to think of these constantly repeated programs as being equivalent to a rut in a road, deepened and broadened with use. On reflection, however, we can see that the system we have described does not call for any such effect. We do not say that the heating system and refrigerator in our homes have the "habit" of turning on at certain temperatures; quite plainly this is the result of biasing, the settings for the purpose. They do not turn on at the present temperature the second or hundredth time any more readily than the first. Just so, the selection of a program from a proster depends on biasing, and in often-repeated settings the biasing tends to be closely similar, so that the same selection results.

In contrast, addressing tends to create ruts simply because more and more clues accumulate. The second time you meet a person, you may have some difficulty recognizing him, but by the tenth time a glance at him or just hearing his voice gives ample clues and the input is far more readily addressed, and categorized down, to produce quick and sure recognition. This can be expressed as a law.

5. Rutting: addressing tends to rut, program selection does not.

If this is correct, we see why the flash of insight or sudden hooking up of two networks occurs so unpredictably and in a chance fashion. In a great variety of teaching situations where insight is sought, the instructor explains and some of the learners understand while others don't, even though apparently they have had ample input. The law above explains this difference. The addressing of the input the instructor offers has rutted, so that it keeps missing the desired connection. Repeating the explanation that didn't work merely deepens the rut, as will slight variations. What is required are very different inputs, or new ones, that will not be addressed right into the old rut.

The back edge of a handsaw in many cases makes an excellent straightedge, and the prong of a hammer may in a pinch serve as a screwdriver. But a worker using these tools may abort a project for lack of a straightedge or a tool to loosen a screw. The saw and hammer are each so strongly addressed, rutted, to their usual applications that they cannot be seen in other lights. Some ingenious experiments have shown how strongly this factor influences behavior.

Does the spontaneous, haphazard firing of neurons act to keep the brain's thinking more flexible? Does it at times, by a purely chance shift of biases or derutting of addressing, produce new connections? The idea is at least fascinating and appears to have a distinct survival value, but by present knowledge this explanation must be regarded as purest speculation. Without depending on chance, how can a changed selection of program be effected, to cope with an ever-changing environment? We can express the answer this way:

6. Change: variation in program selection can be effected (a) by changing bias, and (b) by causing abortion.

If we shift the biases sufficiently—which is to say we perceive the situation differently—the summing procedure of the proster will perhaps lead to selection of a different program (see Figure 10, page 86). There can be many reasons for perceiving the situation differently, including additional input, modification of long-term (frontal) biasing, and those processes often summed up as maturation.

Abortion—the failure of the program to work—can be caused by shifts or changes in the environment, particularly those that are not perceived at all or not appreciated as having importance. A speculator, using certain programs, does well in a rising stock market but loses badly when it begins to drop; a stenographer cheerfully accepts her employer's request for overtime work on a Tuesday but quits when the request is made on a Friday, her day for a date with her new young man; a varnish takes beautifully for an amateur craftsman on a dry, cool day but gives trouble on a damp, hot day. But abortion can be productively applied equally well. To prevent office workers from using an old procedure, for example, the forms previously used are gathered up and destroyed.

To live successfully, we need high flexibility, sensitivity to environment, responsiveness. Because our brain is by evolution a quarrelsome family of three brains, downshifting and upshifting have tremendous effect on how we perceive, think, feel, and act.

7. Threat: in proportion to perceived threat, downshifting to faster, simpler, and more primitive brain function occurs. As a corollary, the less threat and the more confidence is felt, the more effectively the cortex can be utilized.

This law should be considered with reference to the previous one of change, since as a general proposition any downshift is away from fullest use of the newest brain and toward the more change-resistant, traditional, ritualistic brains. By the same token, the faster a decision is made, under pressure, the more certainly a downshift must occur, or at very least a shortcutting of the full cortical processing. Because it has vastly more neurons, the cortex requires far more time to operate at its best. Time pressure, then, may be considered an aspect of threat.

What I have called search represents the most exhaustive use of the cortex. In Freudian terms search would be said to occur in the "subconscious mind," an expression that in my view might best be called quaint. The point is that search is carried on in a nonattentional way, by the planning prosters presumed to be largely in the frontal lobes. Characteristically, search works when, perhaps deliberately, we put our attention elsewhere. Successful use of search involves a specific technique.

8. Search: the procedure is effected by (a) providing strong and specific input, (b) disengaging attention, and (c) avoiding threat and time pressure.

The great bulk of all that man has ever achieved in the way of new ideas, innovation, invention, art, problem-solving, and creativity in general derives from search. This brings us back to the essential nature of the brain, as a comparative-differential analysis device, much more analog than digital, operating by crude approximations rather than precisely, but effecting working accuracy by summing a multiplicity of approximations. It follows that the PAC mode is natural while SSM is artificial.

9. Mode: in proportion to thought process being toward the PAC mode (perception, analysis, choice) and away from the SSM mode (symbol selection and manipulation), thinking is faster, more accurate, effortless, and reliable. Transduction to SSM expression should therefore be the last step, if it must be used at all, for purposes of communication or record or to interface with digital apparatus.

This is simply to say that evolution never designed our brains to push symbols around in precise fashion, and that compared to natural thinking we don't do it well. The common identification of thinking with SSM, or the emphasis on cognitive as superior, more important, more fashionable than PAC mode, reflects first the "logic" brainwashing of formal education; second, ignorance of the nature of human brains; and third, a naive trust in names.

One more law must be added to this list, if only to combat the long years of effort, foredoomed to failure, to understand the brain by fractionation.

10. Totality: the brain functions as a whole, its output reflecting total built-in schemata, stored input, and the summing of total biasing.

Efforts to fractionate the brain have been dictated largely by the convenience of many experimental investigators, who over the years have come to confuse *their* techniques with Psychology. From the techniques grew terminology that snarled them ever more confusedly and unproductively in circular reasoning. But during the same period brain researchers working with nervous systems have made enormous progress, continually finding more and more physical evidence of the unity of the brain in terms of interconnections, switching centers, and diffusion of function. Similarly, those psychologists and others who have taken an ethological or whole-being approach have made rich contributions.

These laws are set forth as major tenets of Proster Theory that hopefully may be tested. For the moment they appear to evidence a general coherence and in many ways fit snugly with much that has been well established, as well as with observations that any of us may make day to day.

PART III

Some Implications and

Applications

CHAPTER 21

How Young Humans Learn

IN THIS concluding section, let us examine some of the implications and applications of Proster Theory.

No more than a small sampling can be attempted, for if this unified model of brain function does in fact give some immediate insights into learning and behavior, the whole range of human activity and inter-relations is opened up to reinspection in this new frame of reference.

For present purposes, the next four chapters will consider briefly how learning begins in infants and youngsters; the disaster we call formal education via conventional schools; the problems and behaviors of adults approached in proster terms; and some thoughts about man's prospects in a complex and increasingly tentative world.

We can begin conveniently with the human infant as it emerges from the womb, creating as a rule a special form of anxiety for its parents. To the best of our knowledge, man is the only species that wonders and worries about how to raise its young. As well we may. The human brain is a superb instrument with the toughness and resilience of a half-billion years of test and development behind it. Yet, more than in any other creature, our brain is open to learn, uncommitted; we have the minimum of built-in circuits. Our neonates are the most completely helpless. Our freak of a brain has staggering potential; but it develops essentially as a device nourished by environment, and if the environment distorts or interferes with its "intended" style of development, lasting trouble can ensue.

The great problem we have in raising children in a highly civilized society derives from the complex, artificial, and largely arbitrary qualities of the environment a family typically lives in. Cause and effect become far separated, even when they are relatively sharply linked. A generator fails in a distant powerhouse, and the child's phonograph will not play. A father disappears for most of the day to his work for reasons totally mysterious to the youngster. Cancellation of a government contract closes a plant and forces the family to move to another city. Incomprehensible hazards surround: electricity in every fixture, gas in the stove, poisons under the kitchen sink, drugs in the bathroom cabinets, matches left on a table, windows to fall out of, fast-moving vehicles in the bordering streets. Without assuming the role of a latter-day Rousseau, one can note the advantages of the simpler times of even grandfather's day, when many children actually saw food grown or gathered and possibly watched a father build some shelves from raw lumber.

The infant born into this most puzzling of worlds has a head far out of proportion to his body to accommodate a brain that already has virtually all its billions of cortical neurons. The neurons must be present because unlike most body cells which constantly die, are replaced, and multiply, neurons just die, at a rate estimated at several thousand a day. (In sixty years, at this pace, the loss would total merely some tens of millions—hardly worth noting; but the rate probably steps up sharply in later life, especially with circulatory impairment. Problems arising from normal attrition seem among the least of our worries.) The head cannot be too big to pass through the birth canal, yet by present knowledge almost all the neurons must be there, ready for development.

Even during gestation, the brain far outpaces the rest of the body. The brain is quite evident when the embryo is scarcely a quarter-inch long! At birth, the brain has reached about 25 percent of its adult weight, while the rest of the body is nearer 5 percent. The brain continues to enlarge rapidly during the first few months of independent life, and faster than the body for several years. At around age five, the brain may be within 10 percent of its ultimate weight, though the head has further to go.

Neurology still has a great deal to learn about the nature of the infant brain. Sufficient knowledge exists, however, to permit saying that in no sense can it be viewed as merely a miniature of the adult organ. Rather it must be regarded as a potential human brain, still very far from organized and physically incomplete in critically important respects. One of these is myelination. The ability of a nerve to conduct impulses is greatly affected by its being wrapped in a kind of insulation provided by what are called Schwann cells. This elaborate wrapping often is segmented, not continuous. Other nerve fibers are insulated by Schwann cells in a different manner. The nature of the insulation, as well as the diameter of the nerves, determines the speed of conduction—the fastest transmit at more than a hundred times the rate of the slowest. Myelination in the cortex goes on for years, probably to about the age at which growth generally comes to a full stop, around twenty. During childhood great areas of cortex have not yet become myelinated. Around the onset of adolescence much of the process, except in the frontal lobes, has been relatively completed; and it may not be coincidental that about age twelve the brain waves, as analyzed by EEG machines and computers, begin to show characteristic adult patterns. The Jewish bar mitzvah ceremony at age thirteen, which marks the passage from childhood to adulthood, may be less arbitrary than it seems.

Myelination was long used as a convenient, unscientific excuse for explaining why reading results should not be expected before age seven or eight. The notion has been blasted: Moore and others have proved beyond doubt that more or less median children can learn to read, and compose prose and verse, as early as three, with enjoyment and profit. In general, children up to early adolescence have been found in recent years to be enormously more capable in many instances that educators previously supposed; under proper circumstances, for instance, eleven-year-olds may romp through "college" mathematics. The myth that students who make such gains don't really move ahead, since others catch up to them, is part of the comforting folklore schools commonly immerse themselves in to avoid confronting the harsh realities of individual differences. Findings of the National Assessment of Educational Progress show that few high school graduates are skillful readers,[1] and several pieces of evidence suggest the great majority of these had a good start on reading before they ever entered first grade.

That learning snowballs is obvious to anyone who will look. An early gain in any significant area means accelerating gains as growth proceeds. We have massive studies that show conclusively, by whatever tests used, that the gap between "slow" and "bright" students widens with each passing year. This is precisely what we would expect if it is true that all learning is built on previous learning; and of course it can be accentuated by differences in input and learning opportunities. It is easier to roll a bigger snowball if you have more access to suitable snow.

We must keep reminding ourselves, when we discuss humans, that one great difference between us and other animals *is* difference. Because we are to such an extreme learning animals, acquiring much of our nature after birth, individuals within the species differ enormously in all ways affected by learning. Particularly as we speak of children, we should also bear in mind that the range of physical variation can be huge. One youngster at sixteen may weigh no more than a heavy child of eight, and a light lad of eight may weigh less than a heavy boy of four. We use the term adolescence, but by various indications the period begins in individuals not at a fairly fixed point but through a range of well over five years. One baby may walk at ten months, another not as well until twenty, yet both must be considered normal. Knowing the age of an individual child and nothing else, we have utterly no precise notion of what he or she looks like, or can do. Even newborn babies show great variation in physique, organization, energy, and what the doctor may call intelligence or apparent alertness.[2]

An infant during its first four weeks usually sleeps most of the time and barely stays awake during the rest. It sucks, yawns, defecates, urinates, makes some slight movements of the limbs, and if male manages a few erections. It also cries. We must beware of saying, or even thinking, that it cries to get some care it requires. Considerable time will pass before this child can do anything whatever "for a reason," in the adult sense. It survives on built-in programs and the attention of adults, who to some degree follow built-in patterns in caring for it. (Let a picture of an appealing baby—whether human, dog, seal, elephant, or panda—come on screen in a movie theatre and a chorus of warm "ahhhs" arises as if a button had been pushed. The schema is so powerful that we tend to be fascinated by almost anything miniature, whether a matchbox model of an automobile, a tiny Bible, or the Bill of Rights on the head of a pin.)

Few transposition thinking efforts are harder than putting ourselves into someone else's skull and seeing the world from the other's point of view. Teachers often pride themselves on being able to get into students' minds to help them get over some difficulty. Undoubtedly, out of thousands of chances, a sensitive teacher does once in a while say or do something that "clicks," and joyously relates the success. As in winning a lottery, a success is worth talking about. Observation and outcomes sadly make it plain that in the vast majority of instances the teacher's effort fails to hit the jackpot, and indeed may serve mainly to make the child feel more frustrated and stupid for not being able to grasp what the teacher, by signals, indicates should be quite clear.

The child's mind is not an adult's on a smaller scale, or on a lower level, or just less experienced. If the work of Jean Piaget has taught us one point above all others, it is this. Not until twelve or so does the brain typically get sufficiently developed physically and (in Proster Theory terms) sufficiently well-stocked with prosters and flexible addressing to function in large part in an adult manner, though the planning-evaluating frontal lobes will still lag far behind.

Consider an infant boy at the age of one month as his eyes follow movement around him—the beginning of a long investigation of this buzzing environment he has been thrust into. In various ways we know rather confidently that the child can distinguish figure from ground, which is to say he does not confuse his mother with the wallpaper behind her, or the side of his bed with the ceiling. He does not follow his mother's movement with his eyes because he is "curious" or even because he knows his mother. The necessity to observe and attend to many kinds of motion is built into our visual system and perseveres until we can no longer see, although we learn to inhibit attention to many familiar movements as time goes on. Also built-in is a preference for looking at something rather than nothing: at a patterned surface rather than a plain one, at objects rather than surfaces. One does not learn much from a flat, plain surface, so there is learning value, hence survival value, in *seeking out* features of the environment. As soon as an infant's brain gets organized enough to permit eyes to track, the aggressive nature of human learning becomes quite evident. The child is born motivated to learn, and will make an effort to find something to learn from.

One of the built-in schemata is an interest in faces, which again seems rather obviously to have survival value. The face seen most will likely be the mother's. She also picks him up, feeds him, changes his diapers, washes him, fondles him. The baby has much more experience of his mother than of his own toes (which he will discover later, with great interest). We must assume at this stage that the child has no way of knowing, so to speak, where he leaves off and his mother begins. This idea may startle us, for as adults we have acquired a very sharp sense of self and of identity; we cannot easily conceive of a human that has not yet learned these limits.

Gradually, over the next few months, the baby will begin to manifest an awareness of objects, and perhaps extend arm and hand. The difference between his own hand and a ball must be *learned*. Somewhere around seven months, by many indications, the infant appears to get the idea that objects have permanence, although it will take more experience for him to master the ins and outs of this strange fact. Again, we have to kick our mental flanks to imagine living in a world in which a ball comes into existence because it has come into sight, and goes out of existence because it has rolled out of sight. In the earliest weeks, this brain does not fret about why phenomena occur. But very soon it will begin to. The great struggle for every child during the years of growth is *to make sense of the world around him*. Learning is not simply additive, gaining more facts, accumulating more experience—although this is the way it is commonly thought of. Rather, it also involves constant accommodation of these inputs so that they make sense and do not offer, *to the child*, obvious mutual conflicts. The process of learning is in important degree one of constantly revising one's grasp of what is going on around one, of how the pieces of this gigantic jigsaw puzzle fit together.

Anyone who rears or works with children gets glimpses of these understandings now and then. The "cute sayings" of children can be revealing if some effort is made to see what they rest on. My own daughter, at three, once asked me if I was rolling up the car windows, at dusk, "so the darkness wouldn't get in." As do many children, she saw the dark as a sort of fluid that inundated the world in the evening. Closing windows, drawing blinds, locking the front door were seen as measures against the dark—a not unreasonable conclusion.

A six-year-old boy believed objects fell because they had "a heaviness" within them, a sort of spirit that pushed them down. He saw a heavy bowl that he feared to carry as pressing down upon the table—as a physicist might see it, though most adults would not. But the idea of the earth attracting the bowl, or of mutual attraction, was totally beyond his grasp, or interest: he did not show any inclination to consider explanations other than "heaviness."

We should distinguish between this kind of rationale and simpler misunderstandings of words—although these can be illuminating too. A little girl in Sunday school inquired in the course of a discussion whether God barked, a query her instructor had no program for coping with. The explanation was ferreted out long after: the family pet was a German shepherd; a psalm often recited stated that "the Lord is my shepherd." The question in this light made perfectly good sense. The incident illustrates the situational nature of much understanding of language.

The understandings or rationales represent, in our terms, complex prosters of the frontal-lobe type, quite apparent chains of thought, sequences of switching, that for convenience can be called evaluation prosters because they have broad application and do not involve specific motor response or overt behavior. At any age, childhood included, individuals do not eagerly give up their beaten pathways of thinking. As many experiments of the game type have shown, a youngster may give the wrong response fifteen or twenty times in a row, before being willing to shift to the new strategy that works. But when the change is effected, typically the new replaces the old fully, and the old type of response is never used again. We may guess that the child simply is defending an established proster until convinced it always aborts (unlike the adult who probably also is concerned to save face and avoid having to revise a considerable related structure of expertise).

The brilliant and exhaustive work of Piaget has given us a firm base for better understanding children's intellectual development. This eminent Swiss psychologist has spent a long lifetime studying real, live children rather than rats, and in normal surroundings, including very detailed observation of his own three offspring. He has written some fifty books, unfortunately in a style far from lucid and difficult to translate. Consequently, it has taken the customary half-century for his basic findings to percolate into American educational attention, and then often in distorted form.

Piaget's ingenious investigation of "conservation" has stood up well under challenge. For the reader unfamiliar with this concept, let us consider briefly some examples. Suppose seven blue counters are laid out in a row. Children up to age six or seven are invited to lay out a matching row of red counters, counting them as they go, in a one-to-one relationship. A child agrees that both rows have the same number of counters. Now the red row is spaced out more widely. The child insists it now has more counters. Or, water is poured from a glass into a tall, thin glass vessel. The child says there is now more water. When it is poured into a low, flat vessel, he says it is not the same amount. Or, seeing a ball of clay worked into some other shapes, he sees the amount of clay as changing. At this stage of development, the child's brain typically cannot yet handle two factors, such as number and length, at the same time. Numerous efforts to teach children conservation have failed. An important point far too little noted, which further underlines our discussion of language, is that the less verbal the adult's effort to teach, the earlier the child shows grasp of conservation. This fits with Piaget's broad finding that the child at this stage learns by *concrete* operations, and also with the Proster Theory view that the child ordinarily does not develop any programs by this age not arising from his own needs. He does not require a grasp of conservation to get along, until adults begin pestering him to do arithmetic—which he cannot do other than by rote until he acquires the expectation that quantity, number, weight, and volume will remain constant despite manipulation. Building these expectations so that they become the end results of programs takes several years. (In fact it has been shown that college students in nonscientific fields may still have a very shaky understanding of why objects sink or float, a more intricate aspect of conservation.)

Just what physical or chemical changes in the brain constitute the process of learning still retains a good deal of mystery. We know that the neuron layers actually thicken, and that RNA appears to play a role, and that the glial cells which surround neurons and probably supply needed materials to the learning process multiply greatly into the realm of hundreds of billions. Many kinds of individual neurons become more complex in extensions and endings. For analogy, we can picture a number of small trees set out in a garden, a few feet apart. As they grow their number does not increase, but their branches and roots intertwine more and more until a virtual tangle develops. Quite literally, a teenager has more brains than a toddler, and quite plainly the *process* of learning produces this kind of brain growth.[3] Maturation presumably sets limits on how fast the development can proceed; but input resulting from varied exposure plays the largest part in bringing about the learning process or changes.

Piaget's work strongly confirms the proposition that all learning must be based on previous learning. Detached learning is not possible: the child can learn only what comes next. Overwhelmingly, Piaget and his associates have shown that the sequence in which children acquire the major concepts rarely varies. As always, however, children differ greatly, and concepts are achieved at a range of rates and ages and at different rates on different fronts. While the learners move through a series of stages, they may advance or lag in particular areas. The assumption that because a child is a certain age he or she is in a certain stage is useful only within gross limits, and can be most misleading when applied to an individual. We can even look at stages as purely an adult view, not anything actually "in" the child.

With this focus on exposure to input, we can more readily see how the brain operates as a comparative-differential analytical device and how learning occurs, from a Proster Theory viewpoint.

The core of learning is the extraction of *patterns* from confusion. This is a lifelong process that begins virtually at birth.

Consider, for example, an infant in its third month of life, and the inputs it may typically receive as its mother and others enter and leave its room or carry it about and care for it. To comprehend the process, we have to attempt to set aside what we know as adults and transpose into the baby's mentality. The table that follows, contrived to illustrate the point, roughly shows the relative frequency of repeated inputs within categories, during a period. (Much of what the infant sees it cannot recognize, save in vague, broad fashion, because it has not yet built recognition programs.)

INPUT	NUMBER OF TIMES
Face, surmounted by large dark area (hair)	xxxxxxxxxxxxxxxxxxxxxxxxxxxxxxxxxxxxxxx
Face, surmounted by small dark area (hair)	xxxxxxxxxxxxxxxxxxxxxxx
Blue area below face (clothes)	xxxxxxxxx
White area below face	xxxxxxxxxxxxxxxxxxx
Red area below face	xxxxxx
Dark area below face	xxxxxxxxxxxxxxxxxxxxx
Long flesh shapes (arms)	xxxxxxxxxxxxxxxxxxxxxxxxxxxxxxxx
Warmth (baby held)	xxxxxxxxxxxxxxxxxxxxxxxx
Pressure on head (held)	xxxxxxxxxxxxxxxxxxxxxxxx
Sucking, food provided	xxxxxxxxxxxxxxxx
Light, intense source	xxxxxxxxxxxxxxxxxxxxxxxxxxxxxxxxxxxxxxxx
Voice sounds, high pitch	xxxxxxxxxxxxxxxxxxxxxxxxxxxxx
Voice sounds, low pitch	xxxxxxxxxxx
Bell sounds (phone)	xx
Light through window	xxxxxxxxxxxxx
Cold, dampness	xxxxxxxxxxxxxxxx

The old idea of association expresses, in one form or another, the relation of two inputs, A and B; if they occur together frequently, they become linked. A glance at the chart, which suggests only a tiny fraction of the inputs raining on an infant, makes plain how hopelessly inadequate this approach is. Never do just two inputs occur together, even for the newborn child, but rather a great many. Some of these, he has to learn, are worthless—as the "area below face" or clothing worn by the person seen may have little or no effect on what happens and changes so often as to confuse rather than inform. Equally, the amount of hair involves misinformation, for at times the mother may enter with hair bound in a scarf rather than falling loose. Learning involves not simple associations but very complex sorting out of patterns, sets of clues that in due course begin to prove reliable (but far from invariable) over the course of hundreds and thousands of trials. The brain apparatus compares similar patterns, matching them against recognition programs that slowly refine from simple and vague (tolerating much deviation) to complex and much more precise (though always tolerating some deviation). It notes differences in similar fashion, and gradually analyzes both negative and positive aspects of comparisons—for example, though the telephone bell is a strong, sharp input, it usually does not affect the child's situation. If the mother is in the room, however, it may, if she leaves to answer the phone. To detect this pattern is, for the baby, a stupendous feat, only possible on the basis of many, many experiences with this set of patterns. Until then, the bell must be analyzed out as what the information scientist calls noise—nonmeaningful input.

If associating A with B were the problem, learning would be rapid. Humans are the slowest-learning animals, in general, because the child must attend to this staggering task of pattern-sorting. To make progress, a huge number of trials is required, which calls for both exposure and time. As the snowball of learning grows, learning speeds up; but we often forget how painfully slow it must be at the outset. As the chart above suggests, the patterns in which frequently, consistently repeated inputs give important information can be learned far faster than those that are more complex and depend on less frequent and less consistent elements. Important means important to the individual infant, not to adults. We know extremely little detail about how recognition programs are built.

The development of motor prosters is much easier to observe, though still difficult to explain. And we note the role of pure repetition. A baby in a highchair who has just learned to release an object so it drops to the floor will do so again and again if he can. Some months later he may pull pots and pans out of kitchen closets, or empty wastebaskets, with the same persistence—until he suddenly stops. We can suspect the proster has been built for the time being. It seems reasonable to assume that recognition prosters similarly are built by repetition, although the child is not as able to control the repeats, and must wait for them to happen.

This throws light on the great desire manifested in early childhood for fixed procedures and rituals. As Caleb Gattegno has shrewdly noted,[4] young children show great interest in television commercials because they do repeat exactly. Much evidence fits together to suggest that repetition may well have a tremendous influence on the child's confidence. The stable home, the loving routines, the bedtime rituals, the consistent parents, all may be essentially important because they involve and permit this factor of exact repetition. As motor or recognition or evaluation prosters become reliable, in terms of outcome—of expectations being realized—the child gains confidence that his inner image of his environment fits his world well enough to enable him to function with a tolerable number of abortions.

In contrast, the child subjected to an excess of abortions because of conflicting inputs, too rapid change, and too little repetition may evidence distress by being overfearful, clinging, withdrawn, aggressive, or hyperactive. Such children, particularly as they reach first grade, may be labeled brain damaged or as suffering from learning disabilities. Children who get far too little input, especially the kind that a loving and capable mother gives, will likely appear retarded.[5]

As many before me have suggested, a child learns much the same way he digests food—the intestines selecting from the input what the body needs. The digestive tract can select, however, only if the input is sufficiently nourishing, and not indigestible or poisonous. For the young child's learning, this appears to translate simply enough as normal attention by adults and exposure to the many activities, things, sounds, smells, and tactile inputs that an ordinary household offers. *People*, providing physical contact, talk, and play, account for the most essential inputs; but television seems an additional source so potent it has helped change the whole calendar for children's achievement.

From this brief venture into a very large area, we can extract the following points as applications of our theoretical approach:

1. From the first month of life on, the child will benefit from pro-

visions of inputs rich in quantity and variety. In general, the more it is exposed to patterns, the faster and better patterns can produce proster formation. Learning snowballs—the more that is learned, the more that *can* be learned as the next layer. But input cannot be force-fed. The child must be free to select its next needs, which seldom are apparent to adults.

2. Repetition plays a major role. The child usually indicates quite clearly when its need for particular repetition ends. Though adult patience can be strained, cheerfully tolerating the child's need seems the obvious part of wisdom.

3. Initial human learning is extremely slow. The child must build on the initial built-in schemata, which are pitifully limited. Even the highly trained and experienced adult has difficulty transposing into the child's mentality. The brain is not a miniature of an adult's, nor one that simply lacks stored knowledge—it is a maturing and developing brain that does not and cannot work in an adult fashion on any level. The child must be allowed to set its own pace and to learn in terms of its own brain at the current stage.

4. The child's comprehensions, or evaluation prosters, grow in an orderly way as it constantly revises its fit with the environment. It can only learn what comes next on any particular learning front: all learning must be built on previous learning. Again, only the individual child knows what comes next, what can now be attached to the snowball. The growth of comprehensions can be encouraged and facilitated by arranging the environment and inputs, but very little if at all by teaching.

The parent who observes the child from a Proster Theory viewpoint, I believe, will much more readily grasp what progress in learning is being made; the building of prosters is often easy to see when one looks for it. And such a parent, respecting a developing brain, may have more success and less frustration in communicating. To tell a typical two-year-old to "stop pulling the tablecloth" will simply encourage it to pull. The sentence is too complex: the "stop" goes one way, the "pull the tablecloth" portion the other. The child responds only to the second part. Change the instructions to "let go of the tablecloth" and results will likely improve. Or better yet, say, "come to me!" with a gesture. The father who tries to teach his four- and five-year-olds some "rules" is wasting his time—they are probably many months away from being able to comprehend an abstract general rule. Nor is it practical to tell preschoolers, "Mother has a headache, so please play quietly." They can't transpose to mother's viewpoint, and even "play quietly" lacks the specifics needed.

With children even more than with adults, reliance on words tends to booby-trap us. We trust them to carry meaning, when actually most of it depends on nonverbal signals and the situation—*the situation as perceived by the child*, which as we have seen differs enormously from that perceived by the adult.

CHAPTER 22

The Assault on the Brain
Called Education

EDUCATION, particularly public schooling, has been criticized and attacked in so many ways during the past fifteen years or so that to offer yet another examination of its grievous faults may seem redundant. But sad to say, the relation of conventional schooling to the brain has been almost totally unexamined. It is not at all easy to find so much as a mention of the word brain in educational literature, especially that small portion commonly seen by the people who operate schools.

We have the absurd circumstance that those entrusted with the "professional" task of educating the rising generation evidence almost total ignorance of how the human brain came to be and how it works. At staggering expense, we engage the blind to lead the sighted. The result, not surprisingly, is a continuing national disaster. That schools are grossly inadequate and in acute trouble is scarcely argued any more: one could not easily find an informed defender of the status quo other than those lamely rear-guarding their own daily efforts, themselves victims of the system and seldom happy with it.

We would expect that people, however earnest, who have no basic understanding of what they are doing would accomplish little in helping to bring about the growth of useful knowledge, skills, and insights. But ignorance is rich manure for myths, and virtually all of us have been brought up with the notion that anything labeled education must be praiseworthy and of value. As in the Sears catalog of old, education came only "good, better, best." The hard thought that schooling might also be discouraging, harmful, or destructive was simply not to be mentioned. This weirdly unrealistic view of schools (millions of parents still hold to it even as they see their own children tortured and cut down to "failures" right before their eyes) has come to feed more and more on *credentialism.* Schooling always serves some distant goal: one goes to elementary school to prepare for middle school, to middle school to get ready for high school, where one must get good credentials in order to go to college, where one must get the required number of "points" to get a degree, which one must have to get a good job, which one must have . . . to make money to send one's children to college? Learning, competency, becoming a confident person able to operate in a complex society and achieve some satisfactions of lasting value—these seem almost brushed aside for the report cards, diplomas, admission to the "right" college, and degrees.

Credentialism is, of course, the polar opposite of interest in and respect for education. Plainly it is not the children who yearn for some ultimate status; only adults can think in such terms. For motives that may range from naive good intentions to blatant using of their children, they join the schools in whipping the student along from goal to goal. Happily, the victims rebel more and more by refusing to yield meekly to pressures. Unhappily, shocking numbers escape by running away, using drugs, dropping out, or attempting suicide.

If we examine the conventional type of school from the viewpoint of Proster Theory, we see that we could hardly devise an environment more perfectly designed to *prevent* learning, cause constant distress, and distort human development.

The class-and-grade school system that most American schools still use dates back more than a century and a quarter. In principle, it has changed very little. Horace Mann, if returned by some time machine for a visit, would recognize it at a glance.[1] It predates almost everything we know about the brain and its workings. A relic from a vanished day, it never served well to produce learning, and today creaks from crisis to collapse as the most expensive absurdity in our society, a continuing assault on the brains of the hapless and trusting children forced to attend. The kind of school in which curriculum is prepared in advance, and then taught, is basically harmful. Some children manage to escape much damage, but many more are permanently harmed, and an intolerable number suffer what amounts to psychological butchery. These last include predominantly the poor and those who are "different" by color or language, but we should not lose sight of the studies that find the most able students among the chief victims.[2]

The subject cries out for full examination, but here we can note only the most obvious horrors and insanities, in Proster Theory terms.

1. Learning is inhibited by threat, since threat produces down-shifting. Threat pervades the conventional school. It begins with *captivity*, itself a direct threat going to the deepest roots of evolutionary history—for eons, captivity, lack of freedom to move, was equivalent to quick and painful death, or a slower end by starvation. The school makes the child captive within a building, then within a room, and, when assigned seating is used, within various strange kinds of desks that even look like traps. We do not literally chain the student in place, but the effect is much the same: the child cannot move two feet without permission or penalty.

Fear is what makes the great majority of present schools run. By second or third grade almost all children have learned how the system works. Whether the teacher be kind or harsh matters little, for the ultimate choice is simple and clear: the student will comply and conform, or punishment will be applied, increasing in degree as required. The extreme can involve physical beatings (still approved by the majority of teachers),[3] suspension, or expulsion. Most often the club is simply the report card or the note sent home, usually enough to bring the parent down on the child jointly with the school. Ever present, too, are the psychological beatings of ridicule, sarcasm, shaming before a peer group, or embarrassment—the fear of being laughed at respects neither ability nor social level. In no class that operates as a group can any student feel sure that some crushing put-down is not more than moments away.

Imagine that in an office or factory each worker knew that any error might promptly be announced by loudspeaker for all to hear. Few adults could stand such an arrangement for even a month. The child in a classroom operates under far worse threat, for years on end.

Most of those who operate schools prefer to deny that pervasive fear exists (not all—some like to boast of how they "keep the kids in line"), yet almost any teacher will concede that many of his students will not readily participate in discussion, or display imagination in any effort, or risk any venture on their own, even a mild joke. The student who is not afraid, who challenges, questions, risks unusual answers or original work, usually learns soon enough that such tactics don't pay. Since they in effect threaten the all-important teacher's control, the child must sooner or later be slapped down as "bright, but too fresh."

Downshifting did not bother the classroom type of school or its even harsher precursors so long as emphasis remained on the standard rote right answer. Fear does not prevent the memorization of catechism. But as schools turned more and more from the inadequacies of rote responses and sought much more complex intellectualizing, fear and learning came into head-on conflict. Threat shortens and hurries the process of perception, limits addressing to the most obvious channels, and reduces search to a minimum. In sum, *under threat we cannot use most of our brain power*. The typical classroom, based on captivity and incessant threat, can hardly be surpassed as a counterproductive environment.

2. We have examined the PAC and SSM modes of thinking. So far as the conventional school is concerned, the PAC natural way of thinking scarcely gets recognition, and when detected is promptly squashed. As a host of critics point out, the present type of school tends to be obsessed with evaluation, in primitive and arbitrary ways, of almost everything the student does. Each response, test, essay, report, homework task, and formal examination gets scored and often recorded in a Domesday Book. A student soon learns that giving expected responses will make life in school more tolerable, and that following the approved logical procedures and forms will more likely win better evaluation (marks). Not much later, he or she discovers that marks are what count, not learning—good marks get approval and reward in school and at home and ultimately may provide entry to the right college and perhaps graduate school. A youngster must be either foolish or a maverick not to play the game of pleasing the teacher, one way or another, as the issuer of the interminable evaluations.

Most teachers love marks. Despite the protests they may offer, claiming that parents demand them, it seems evident that the power to give marks constitutes the core of the teachers' control, and is the last aspect of the old classroom they willingly surrender. SSM procedures lend themselves readily to the kind of evaluation used for marking. But PAC thinking doesn't, and its outcomes can be disturbing, even frightening, to the teacher clinging to group control of the class. Consider the student who, during work on long division, invents by PAC a different algorithm for the same purpose. The rare teacher may exult at the achievement; but far more likely the inventor will be told, "We don't need new methods. Do it the way I'm telling you, and don't confuse things." The teacher has a point: life will be easier for him or her if the official algorithm is used, rote fashion. But the effect is to suppress the PAC intuitive problem-solving type of thinking that has produced virtually all of mankind's artistic and intellectual achievements!

The natural, fast, easy, enormously efficient PAC mode gets suppressed in the classroom school in part for this reason of control, but perhaps even more because, in their own education, school people have been thoroughly brainwashed into believing that only *what can be put on paper* is respectable. As we have seen, PAC approaches using search cannot be explained. The engineer or manager or scientist who solves a problem by hunch, or by having the answer suddenly pop into his head while bathing, literally does not know how the solution was produced by the brain. The lad "stupid in arithmetic" who catches the ball in the playground clearly has a brain that works expertly in this respect, but since symbol manipulation on paper is not involved, the achievement is brushed aside.

To comply with the classroom demands, the student must put his symbols on paper, and even then in conventional, rote, accountable ways, in which "logical" procedures are evident. One is reminded of the Chinese court ladies whose feet were bound in their youth until by adulthood they could only hobble. By systematically suppressing and penalizing PAC approaches, the school with rare exception binds the natural capacities of the human brain so far as it can.

Evaluation by marking is, of course, one more aspect of threat. So we find an ironic conflict created by the school as it attempts to use for the teaching of symbol manipulation an organizational structure designed for rote learning. The use of symbols in this manner is exceedingly difficult and counter to natural brain function —somewhat like trying to force an analog computer to behave in digital ways. Yet ability to use SSM approaches where properly called for is essential to today's educated person, and manifestly seems one goal for schooling. But we find that in mathematical reasoning, the most common form of SSM instruction, the schools fail most miserably, even more than in reading. Much of the explanation seems plain: the SSM effort in the classroom is subject to constant evaluation, which means constant threat, which produces constant downshifting, which makes SSM thinking (requiring fullest use of the cortex) all but impossible. SSM effort and evaluation clash head-on.

3. In the conventional classroom where the teacher aggressively "teaches," activity tends to be extremely verbal, and despite the ultimate goal of words on paper, heavily oral. Words, words, words are in use most of the day; but up to 80 percent of the time, the teacher dominates the talk, not the students. Indeed, "stop talking" is the commonest injunction to the students. Kept silent, talk-deafened, they are periodically tested on their skill with the words they have been systematically prevented from using![4]

If the teacher's lecturing and exposition conveyed a great deal of information, it might be expected to accomplish some learning. But here the "words-have-meaning" booby trap takes a heavy toll. Teacher talk may have very little situational content to the students —far less than to the adult using them. The teacher has the illusion of giving copious information and enlightenment, says "I taught," and cannot understand why the students have not learned in proportion. The first reaction is to blame the students for their dullness and inattention, the second to repeat the same nonsituational effort that failed the first time—now called review.

While this exercise in mutual frustration goes on endlessly, the teacher does give out a stream of nonverbal signals that the students receive very effectively. These tell the youngsters what response the teacher wants. At the chalkboard, for example, asking whether an equation is right or wrong, the teacher may signal by posture, motion, facial expression, or tone of voice which answer the class should give. For survival under threat, learning to interpret such signals has obvious value, and children become very adept at parroting back answers the teacher's unaware behavior tells them is desired. They haven't learned, but they give right answers. Or, struggling for them, they ignore talk and watch for signals.

To teachers aggressively instructing groups, response becomes essential as permission to proceed to the next point or step. Failure to get it forces some form of repetition of the teaching effort that apparently hasn't succeeded. As with any other abortion, distress results; the teacher wants evidence of learning, wants to move ahead. To give out ample nonverbal signals, then, is to make teaching seem easier. To further insure responses, teachers working in conventional classrooms typically confine almost all their attention to eight or nine students, usually located front and center, who can and do oblige with the responses wanted. (Teachers vigorously deny such behavior, but evidence shows their impression of their own work differs sharply from the observation of third parties.) Visiting any such classrooms, one is likely to observe within the first two minutes a teacher accepting a response as though it meant that all the class understood.

4. This emphasis on words and symbols, with its implication that respectable or important thinking must be in such terms, combines with the captivity factors to make the school the haven of nonreality. The walls not only keep the students in, but the real world out. Visit many classrooms of a conventional school system, with reality/nonreality in mind. It soon becomes apparent that most rooms provide enclaves, sterile to an extreme, in which the great majority of objects are concerned with *representations* of reality: words, symbols, maps, charts, diagrams, pictures, and associated apparatus (much of which the students may not freely touch or use). When we bear in mind the import of Piaget's work, particularly as it affects the lower grades, we see how utterly, desperately inappropriate the environment is. Real objects, real materials, real problems are essential for intellectual development in the child up to age twelve or so, and highly desirable for older students as well.

Being restricted to representations and abstractions rather than reality, and to the prissily filtered input of the schoolroom rather than real society, raises effective barriers to useful learning. But there is a worse penalty, which is perhaps more readily visible in the light of the proster approach. The importance of fit between inner image and outer environment has been examined. The test of the inner image is the realistic success of the proster based on it, when used within the environment. The answer—this program works, or aborts —*comes from the environment*. For example, a child of five tries to put a nut onto a bolt. If he holds both pieces correctly and turns them the right way, the nut goes on, otherwise it will not. An older girl, skipping rope, finds out *from the rope* whether she has the skill to go through an elaborate routine. In each case the real environment renders the decision.

But in the classroom school, the rules suddenly change. The decision now comes overwhelmingly from one source—the teacher. What the teacher says is good is good, what is wrong is wrong, what is inadequate is inadequate. Answers cease to come from real sources. Learning by detecting patterns and constant testing of the environment and percepts gives way to pleasing an all-powerful master. To make matters worse, the teacher is not too likely to say "wrong" to a favored student as bluntly or in the same tone as to one disliked or considered inferior. It has long been known that liked students get higher marks for just that reason.

The difference can be devastating. Seeking the answer to fit directly from real circumstances, the learner feels it to be wholly or largely impersonal. When the basketball misses the hoop, the player says, "I shot it wrong." But when classroom answers are declared wrong by the teacher, with frequency, the child probably will in time conclude, "There is something wrong with me *as a person.* I am inferior, hated, despised, or rejected." Forced to attend school to suffer this daily torture, the student responds with the despondency of hopelessness, withdrawal, hate, or perhaps violence expressed in vandalism or the street crime we so loudly lament. (Most of such crime is committed, as F.B.I. periodic reports plainly reveal, by youngsters of school age or just beyond—an uncomfortable fact often ignored.)

5. The role of addressing, as we have seen, is crucial both in perception (the input must be addressed to the correct recognition proster) and in retrieval, via what we call memory or by the process I have called search. In the classroom where evaluation constantly goes on, addressing becomes distorted. Youngsters seldom take much genuine interest in goals many years remote, such as going to an Ivy League college or getting a job with a prestigious engineering firm. The younger the student, the more today and tomorrow take precedence; and a child must be dull indeed not to see that learning is for the purpose of giving a right answer in class, now, or getting by a test next week, or doing well on a major examination next month.

Why does the student learn how to calculate the circumference of a circular cylinder from its radius? Is he planning to make use of some cylinders? Or has he in mind that Mr. McCabe, his teacher, will soon ask the question on a quiz?

Confined to classrooms concerned largely with nonreal problems, the student addresses this bit of learning, temporarily memorized, not to cylinders but to Mr. McCabe's questions. When some weeks later he escapes Mr. McCabe, presumably permanently, any learning retained becomes like a document lost in the files. It is there, but the means of retrieval has for practical purposes been lost: the addresses "school," "final examination," "Mr. McCabe," "room 202," "third period," "textbook" are no longer useful. A year later, working on a problem of wrapping a band around an actual cylinder in the course of building a model, the idea of using the formula will probably not occur to him—he has never used such mathematics for his own purposes!

Day after day and year after year such learning as does occur is systematically misaddressed. To make matters worse, the whole range of human knowledge is absurdly chopped up by educators into subjects and courses and units, and then taught in a fixed sequential way that makes learning and addressing by patterns—the basic brain way of functioning—as difficult as possible. The interconnections, the multiplicity of pathways that make the stored resources of the brain available, are quite deliberately prevented in the interest of academic and administrative convenience.

Considering these five criticisms, one might conclude that if Proster Theory has reasonable validity, the conventional type of eggcrate schools with classes "managed" by teachers must produce extremely little learning, as well as harming great numbers of children in the process. This, of course, is just what we do find, once we forget the nobility of education and the joys of credentialism, and commence to look at the *results* of schooling with eyes fully open.

We do not have to doubt that children learn during the period of a dozen or more years of schooling. The question must be whether they learn materially (or are impeded or mislearn) by exposure to the schools' routine. Today our children are born into a world that has a high information input level—but to attend school means to spend 10,000 waking hours in a generally lower, often impoverished input climate! The presentation of information, ideas, and relationships in the ordinary classroom goes painfully slowly and primitively, and the input of patterns so vital to most learning gets virtually neglected, since there usually will be no understanding of the need. The question we must ask, in all seriousness, is whether the school is facilitating learning, or impeding and distorting the process.[5]

To determine the broad results of classroom instruction, we need (1) to establish a base, the student's knowledge and grasp at the beginning of the instruction; (2) make comparable tests at the end of the unit of instruction so that any differences can be observed; and (3) retest after a lapse of a year or more, since learning is universally distinguished from temporary remembering. The tests used, of course, need to deal with important aspects of the learning aimed for—but most tests used in the schools deal not with what is important but *what is easiest to test*. They tend to be heavily fact or content oriented, concerned with right answers that usually can be readily memorized without much understanding.

When we look at what schools commonly *do*, we find virtually no use of pretesting. Suppose a classroom teacher does pretest, and finds that four of the students know the material very well, and five more could get a passing grade—what on earth is she to do with these youngsters while she teaches the unit? On the other hand, if she does not pretest, and finds at the end of the unit that these nine students score well on tests, she can take credit for their having learned. Teachers, being human, take the sensible and easy way out. To pretest is to make trouble for oneself. Why do it?

The tests used after the unit are overwhelmingly what may be called the regurgitation type. At all levels, including college, students' dominating problem is "what will be asked on the finals?" Teachers who indicate likely questions are considered fair, those who don't are in the students' eyes unfair, sneaky, or treacherous.

From the instructors' viewpoint, one must comply with the social-structure demands of the institution. It does not do to have the students score too well (this indicates the teacher may be "soft"), or too badly (which might suggest that the teacher is not very good, or is mean, or is "hurting students' records"). Both testing and scoring are therefore manipulated to obtain outcomes that are polite and customary within the context of the institution in which, afer all, the instructor has to survive and earn a living. As educational literature endlessly suggests, the whole business of giving exams and grades is tragic, farcical, ritualistic, senseless, deplorable. But in education those are hardly urgent reasons to stop doing anything.

The third requirement, the "longitudinal" testing, is more thoroughly ignored even than pre-testing. Schools have not the slightest motive to find out whether learning was retained. To find out that it wasn't (as is too often obvious) would simply be one more embarrassment—particularly if this third round of testing were not "right answer" in character, but rather asked whether the student *used* the knowledge or learning in any productive and successful way. Such testing would shatter the school's pretensions. We have a mass of evidence[6] that millions of high school graduates cannot read with much skill (sometimes not at all, for practical purposes), nor do simple arithmetic reasoning, nor speak a foreign language with any facility in conversation, nor solve a simple scientific problem, nor write a paragraph of decent expository English, nor explain how legislation goes through Congress or their state legislatures. When we consider that such students have devoted some 10,000 hours to instruction in such matters, over a period of ten or twelve years, we must indeed marvel.

When we look at the other side of the coin, at students whose conspicuous achievement is shown not by marks but by exceptional command and advanced progress, we almost always find that their success was *not* attributable to the classroom, where they obviously did not fit into the group. Rather, they did most of their learning on their own, probably beyond the school. If a teacher helped, it was probably outside the usual classroom routine and schedule.

Very slowly, with exquisite pain, we are coming as a nation to realize the once incredible: that our vaunted school system, however it has served us in the past (a matter of sharp debate), is today a gigantic hoax. It waves the gleaming banner of education while in fact its rituals accomplish almost no learning. On balance the class-and-grade type of school, whether in slum, rural area, or posh suburb, must be judged overwhelmingly harmful and destructive.

We agonize publicly about the drug problem, about "crime in the streets" and burglary. We should also agonize about incredibly rampant venereal disease, second in incidence only to the common cold. We deplore alienation, anomie, the lowering of standards, the deepening disbelief and distrust evidenced by youth. (In the 1972 elections, in which millions aged eighteen to twenty-one were able to vote for the first time, fewer than half went to the polls.) But we keep looking everywhere but at education for explanations, despite massive, hard evidence available that these problems are anchored and fostered in our schools.

Is it wrong to blame the schools for everything? Clearly one can go too far; other influences exist. But no other compares with the schools, attended by almost every child, usually for a dozen years. Those of us of older generations may fail to reflect on how heavily pressures to "get a good education" bear on today's child—the goal being credentials, paper passports which in fantasy will ensure success and the good life. For a girl, good marks may even be stressed by parents so that she can enter a "better" college and so acquire a husband of higher standing, suitably credentialed for generous earnings.

On one hand, the child spends years in institutions that every adult seems to say are of tremendous importance and benefit. On the other, only the dullest student can fail to see the school as usually a dismal factory, infinitely boring save for friends, social activities, sports, and the daily game of beating the system. Schools give education a bad name. And since schools are seen by youngsters as being "official" society, society fails to win much admiration either. The youngster who is labeled a failure by the school may well conclude that only in some counter society can he or she hope for any achievement or reward. As many studies consistently show, the school literally drives great numbers of students into crime, rackets, prostitution, alienation in some form, or the hopelessness so characteristic of persistent poverty.[7]

But even these negative effects pale in comparison with the deadly damage done by persuading the child not to use his brain, to distrust its natural functions, to believe that only symbol manipulation counts —and then setting every obstacle in his path to learning this manipulation.

For a dozen interminable years the conventional school, in its ignorance of the human brain, does almost everything wrong, and then blames society for the problems it generates or aggravates.

Should we have schools at all? It seems to me we need learning centers more today than ever. But each day we retain the antibrain kind of class-and-grade school that we generally have is one too many. What should we have?

Proster Theory focuses on learning. It does not automatically provide a theory of instruction, and certainly not a theory of teaching in the usual sense, since it indicates that aggressive teaching will likely do more harm than good. But the theory does, as a useful learning theory should, strongly suggest some of the basic requirements for successful schools. The key ones are:

1. Freedom from threat.
2. Reality principle.
3. Respect for natural thinking.
4. Communications emphasis.
5. Manipulation emphasis.
6. Addressing for use.
7. High input for pattern learning.

Freedom from threat requires not merely kindly teachers and gentle administrators, but totally expunging every vestige of the class-and-grade system, which is built on threat and incorporates captivity in its very structure. The test for threat is not what the adults say, but how the students feel as shown particularly by how they behave.

The converse side of the requirement is perhaps the greatest single factor in successful learning: the building of confidence in the learner, especially when the learner is a child or youth. Dr. Jerome Kagan, professor of human development at Harvard University, has observed that "One of the few sound principles possessed by psychology is that individuals will cease investing effort in a problem if they doubt their ability to solve it—if they have no expectation of success."[8] The importance of confidence, self-esteem, has come forward again and again, in a great variety of experimental approaches, including the now impressively buttressed Pygmalion effect (expectations producing matching results, either negative or positive),[9] and the spectacular achievements of Moore.

Confidence seems to rest not simply in a belief that the learner can cope, but more fundamentally in trust, resulting from experience, that one or more failures will not result in being demeaned, losing love or regard, or being at least to a degree thrust out of the group—a fear that goes far back in man's social history.

Some families build confidence in children by consistent respect for the child as a person, rather than a chattel or nuisance. (When permissiveness reaches the point of conveying to the child a lack of concern, it becomes a rejection.) Other parents demand compliance and conformity; *not* being a person, an individual, a human with the right to be different. Their punishment of the child will likely be frequent, quick, physical, and sometimes vicious. But evidence indicates that even children so treated can find a haven in the school, if as rare exception it does not provide more of the same. The rather sudden flowering of such children, as they discover they belong not among the despised but with "those who can," has almost a miraculous quality.

Reality principle simply means that the tasks students engage in, the materials they use, and the settings they enter should be real rather than contrived, attenuated, and distorted for curriculum purposes. In the early grades, for instance, the books most frequently used are for teaching reading. No child in his right mind would ever read some of them for content or pleasure. Soon the child works endless problems in arithmetic, contrived for practice. Later, students may perform scientific "experiments" that are merely exercises, the outcomes foregone and already in print. Education is seen not as doing but as preparing.[10] It would make as much sense to lecture children on swimming for years, but never let them enter water. Reality principle lets the right answer come from actual materials or circumstances rather than in words of judgment or evaluation from a teacher. (This is not identical with "learning by doing," which may or may not be realistic.)

Respect for natural thinking, the use of the brain in PAC mode, does not imply discarding SSM methods where they are useful or required. The entire PAC–SSM continuum needs accommodation, with recognition that PAC is the natural, much more frequently productive mode.

Communications emphasis links to reality principle. Most of the use of language in conventional schools, amazingly, does *not* involve any genuine communication. Teachers most of the time talk *at* the students, as one might talk into a microphone with no assurance an audience listens. Most of what students write does not communicate, but is merely an exercise to be evaluated. Students commonly give up trying to talk to teachers because they find they are not listened to, are not understood, or are betrayed; and the classroom constantly discourages talking to one another. Yet what can be a more essential part of development as a human than acquiring skill in giving and receiving communications? Genuine two-part communication represents both essential skills and the prime means of learning about the world we live in.

Manipulation emphasis brings us into a fascinating area that can be no more than mentioned here. In a sense, threat is involved. Does a child feel that reading, or arithmetic, is some kind of unfathomable, ritualistic beast that can devour him, or merely materials, relationships, that *he* can push around? Once a student becomes aware of the power to manipulate (often by PAC approaches), confidence wells up, and the doors to learning open. Much conventional teaching discourages manipulation, at levels right up through the doctorate!

Addressing for use rather than for answering the teacher's questions and examinations, needs no further discussion. This too ties in, of course, with reality principle.

High input for pattern learning is perhaps the need least met by schools, even the more advanced. Learning, as we have seen, depends essentially on pattern recognition, which in turn depends on high input, with much repetition and minor variation. The open, informal classroom, so advantageous in many respects, fails badly as a rule in this.[11] In schools of all kinds, characteristically, input is low and a great deal of the time there is no input at all—a staggering amount of time goes for organizing, ceremonies, movements, arrangements, or disciplining, with nearly zero value in input that could contribute to learning. The stupefying boredom that blankets most schools attests this lack, but we also observe that for most students in a classroom, much of the time, nothing is happening. *Waiting* is a major use of time.[12]

If schools generally are as antibrain as I have indicated and fail badly as a consequence, how is it that they continue? Why have they so broadly resisted changing under the intensive attacks and storms of criticisms of the past dozen years? How can we suffer, as citizens or parents, the tightly organized, legalized, credentialized assault upon our children without feeling, to use the famous phrase of Alfred North Whitehead, "a savage rage"?

This complicated question requires an even more intricate answer, ramifying too far to be fully attempted here. Just a few of the main elements may be noted:

1. The schools compose a vast, interwoven bureaucracy, involving government at many levels; a ragged body of laws, regulations, and taxing powers; parents, taxpayers, and students with conflicting interests; the colleges and universities who profess to train teachers and administrators (a major source of income for many); the outworn board of education control device; the publishers of textbooks and other materials; an enormous variety of suppliers; the designers and builders of schools. This hodgepodge of vested interests is larded over with, currently, a $60-billion expenditure each year, in elementary and secondary public funds alone. The inertia of this shapeless mass seems to prove overpowering.

2. Parents, who could by even a small amount of coordinated "savage rage" create an effective force for major change, all too often function as participants in the essential fraud: the pretense that education is the prime concern of the schools, when actually custody is the dominant role. In John Holt's vivid words, they serve as "day jails"[13] to keep students out of the home, off the streets, out of sight, and out of jobs. As one who has labored in the vineyard, I can testify to how few parents in a community, at any income or educational level, ordinarily take an interest in what goes on in schools. Most, I deeply suspect, do not want to know—for that might mean taking back at least some of the custody and services they pay taxes to have the schools perform.

3. In common with some other prosperous countries, we have come far on the road to being a nation of child haters. Children were once economic and household assets. In large families they were easier to care for; there were grandparents, aunts and uncles, older

siblings, and a community of neighbors, as well as more room. But children have become staggering liabilities financially: it can cost around $80,000 to bring a middle-class child from birth through college.[14] Just as bad, perhaps, is the endless conflict that has come to be associated with child-rearing, including the uncertainties, guilt, and arguments that afflict parents. Hardly surprising is the plunge in the birth rate as means of contraception and abortion become more available. While birth rates tend to fluctuate for complex reasons, certainly we face the possibility that over a period the rate could drop well below zero growth, to a form of gradual, and not necessarily slow, national suicide.

4. But the overwhelming reason we put up with our schools, I believe, brings us back to the core of this book: programs and prosters. People know the schools need sweeping change but do not know what to change *to*. New, alternative programs that would add up to change sweeping enough to be meaningful have not yet been coherently put forward.

Nor are the old programs easy to drop, even under stress. Examined in Proster Theory terms, we see only too plainly that they are not only deeply rutted, but entrenched further by being tied to certification. A teacher who executes a group of approved programs thereby becomes acceptable and may gain a place on the payroll and perhaps tenure. (A present fad is "performance-based" hiring of teachers, who must exhibit ability to perform the orthodox programs, even though there is almost total lack of evidence that the resulting behavior has any relation to producing learning.) For the teacher on the job who would attempt significant change from the established ritual, the innumerable, insistent biases of the setting tend to be overwhelmingly resistant. The organization of the school, the conservatism of many parents and of school boards, the tangle of laws and regulations at many levels, the form of the budget, and the pressures of the classroom setting itself all tend to force teachers into using programs that fall well within the ritual limits. Performing the ritual in orthodox fashion keeps one on the payroll, regardless of results.

Nor can we safely assume that the parents, taxpayers, board of education members, and legislators who influence our schools all *want* to produce graduates who more fully use their brainpower in a confident and individual (and perhaps nonconformist) way. The fourth annual Gallup Poll on Public Attitudes toward Education,[15] for example, showed that getting better jobs, making more money, and getting along better with people ranked far above all other objectives. As in the previous polls, intellectual and cultural achievement scored at the very bottom, conformity and proper behavior at the top.

Anyone who has worked some length of time in community school affairs becomes well aware of the rigidity of programs that the older part of the population displays. The speeches at public meetings, on either conservative or progressive side, sound almost prerecorded. Only as parental biases also change, and permit the choice or building of new programs, can we hope for more than scattered change to modernize our schools.

Fortunately, the biases seem to be changing. Education is less trusted as the automatic conveyor to success. Students instead increasingly see it as a means of making them like their parents— a goal which many likely reject rather than unquestioningly accept. As expenses soar, in taxes and college costs, harder questions are asked by those who must pay. Declining population forces painful reappraisals. Although many parents still don't realize it, the competition to enter college that caused so many to literally sweat over their children's school record has given way to a shortage of students that has many admissions officers scrambling, in some cases begging for applicants. In sum, these are substantial shifts in biases, and they open the way for new programs to actuate the behavior of those who affect the course of schooling.

To this we can add the growing realization that well-funded foundation efforts, and the enormously expensive Office of Education federal programs, have produced only occasional encouraging results, among more evident disasters.[16] In the much publicized report *Inequality*, Christopher Jencks and associates stated: "We can see no evidence that either school administrators or educational experts know how to raise test scores, even when they have vast resources at their disposal."[17] The old faith that lack of funds was the problem, that money could buy education, has suffered rude blows.

The "brain approach" to schooling and education in general may then have one virtue of importance: it is new. It is mired not in the failures and politics and frustrations of the past, nor in the more recent outpouring of billions that have proved again how seldom direct attacks on problems, rather than a sound theory-based effort, have appreciable effect.

The concept of brain-compatible schools not only opens new doors, but presents many handles that we can grasp for almost immediate application—at least to create exemplary, pilot units that can escape old biases and programs, and demonstrate their worth, let us hope, by results achieved. To the best of my knowledge, this inviting approach has had virtually no investigation, no support, no funding whatever—not a thousandth part of one percent of the vast sums annually expended; and has yet to win the attention of those able and persistent leaders within education whose efforts achieve what small gains are being made.

Can our existing schools be converted to brain-compatible practices? Over the past several years, with the help and support of my associate, Dr. Maurie Hillson of the Rutgers Graduate School of Education, and others, I have labored on design of a system that might use much of the present plant, structure, and staff to this end, utilizing and integrating a long list of innovative techniques well known to be at least workable. The resulting "blueprint," known as IROSS (Infinitely Responsive Open School System), has not yet been translated into operation as a whole. But that such a plan can be constructed even on paper seems significant: it suggests that the parts may well be already available, awaiting assembly in the light of a guiding theory that can indicate with some reasonable reliability what to do and what not to do, and that contains provision for the essential retraining of staff.

Donald Snygg, a prominent educational psychologist, has neatly stated the need for theory:

> Knowledge of what has happened in one situation cannot, without a theory of why it happened, enable us to predict what will happen in any other situation if it is different in the slightest degree. If we cannot predict the results of our acts we cannot choose between alternative courses of action or plan new ones.[18]

No theory, however sound, will much influence the three million people working in or with schools who can commence their professional work, carry it on, have their pay raised year after year, and retire on pension, without ever requiring an inkling of what a theory really is and how one is utilized. But general reeducation is hardly the first goal. Among the three million are a few thousand, more sophisticated, who do grasp that we live in a world dominated by theory, and who hunger for principles they can *use*. Hope, I think, lies in a brain-based theory serving as a guide to these leaders and boat-rockers—many of them of impressive ability—to create pilot schools, institutions that for the first time in man's history will not reflect folklore, ritual, and cut-and-try, but will be rationalized, coherent environments designed for the society we are in, not one that has disappeared.

Even a few such learning centers, achieving some striking results, might attain wide influence.

CHAPTER 23

Living with Your Own
and Others' Prosters

Does Proster Theory give us a means of understanding more clearly, and even to some extent predicting, the behavior of humans we deal with—including ourselves?

I would suggest that it does. Yet we must quickly note that a theory of learning and a theory of behavior are not the same, but overlap to a large extent—since much human behavior is wholly or largely learned.

Our behavior is influenced, for example, by a large range of in-body factors. How an individual behaves will likely be affected by whether he feels fresh or tired, is hungry or digesting a heavy meal, feels in excellent health or sick, or needs or has had refreshing sleep. Generally such factors have very little learned content. At the other extreme are largely unlearned species-wisdom factors, genetically transmitted, that we know all too little about, but that are finally being more adequately investigated. They probably influence behavior broadly and continually.

Between these we can easily detect ambient factors. Hot sun, good or bad air, high humidity, heat or cold, heights, colors, lighting, and noise all influence behavior. We can extend *ambient* to the general circumstances we are in: we may respond differently to a film when seeing it in a crowded theater than when seeing it in an almost empty one, or feel a sense of alarm in wind and dark that we would not have in the same place in bright daylight.

When we send pioneers into space or to live for weeks deep under water, such ambient factors are likely to be given close attention. But ordinarily, conventional psychology, with its emphasis on stimulus and experiments with relatively simple animals in deliberately simplified circumstances, tends to throw us sharply off the track. To understand humans better, we need to see them as highly complex creatures attacking and coping with, as well as responding to, very complex and rapidly changing settings and events that typically involve other humans.

As no other creatures do, humans behave in the present but carry with them, as invisible baggage, a large amount of past and a sizeable bundle of future. How we deal with settings and events depends on our individual past, as stored in the brain; on our image of ourselves, which—including plans, aims, expectations—falls largely into future; and on our present state, affected by in-body and ambient factors.

In brief, the worst mistake we can make in trying to gain insight into human behavior is to look for and accept explanations that are too simple. Yet almost everywhere we see people trying to influence or control other people on the basis of absurdly simple causes or remedies. We tell people not to litter or park or come late or drop clothes on the floor, that they should be kind to customers, keep phone calls short, use seat belts, and mail early in the day; we warn them of the consequences of smoking and the penalties for committing crimes—often with little or no visible results, or perhaps even with negative outcomes.

The great bulk of interactions among people fall readily into three general categories:

1. Efforts to get another party to change behavior or do something new.
2. Efforts to mesh behaviors of two parties so that they do not conflict but coincide or become mutually tolerable.
3. Efforts to begin or carry on mutually supportive activity.

Examples of the first could be mother's attempt to get Johnny to wipe his muddy feet before entering the house, a young man's campaign to get a girl to notice him, a woman's volunteer work to win votes for a bill she wants passed. For the second, we can turn to any married couple and observe the minor struggles over which program to watch on television or whether the bedroom window should be open or closed. For the third, we can again consider the bedroom, or the innumerable mutually supportive daily activities of office, shop, factory, laboratory, or of team play.

These categories are listed in order of the trouble they give rise to. Effecting change can be highly frustrating and productive of stubborn resistance or strong emotions. Efforts to mesh or adjust behavior typically produce testiness, argument, and minor quarrels. At the third level, matters go much more smoothly, at worst bringing low-key grumbling or marginal annoyance. If we examine the three categories again in the light of prosters, we see that the first calls for aborting old prosters or building new ones—not efforts to be undertaken casually if favorable results are expected. The second does not call for proster building, but rather for terminating the program in use. If the program, rather than being more or less voluntarily turned off or modified by its user, is indeed aborted, fireworks become likely. Pull out the plug of a radio someone is listening to, or shout "Stop that instantly!" and the abortion must produce emotion. We can even define tact as, to a large extent, a technique for relatively *slowly* turning off the program in use. Consider the wife who calls to her husband after dinner:

"Dear, are you watching television?"

"Yes, I'm watching the game."

"Oh."

"Why, you want something?"

"Well, maybe, when you come to a commercial, would you take out the garbage?"

Some years ago, while vacationing in Vermont, I had occasion to make some purchases at a tiny crossroads store. The first few times, I hurried in, stated what I wanted, put my money down, and left as soon as served. It dawned on me, however, that my city ways were not making me a popular patron. The next time, I entered slowly, ambled my way to the counter while inspecting various merchandise and notices, exchanged a remark or two on the weather, and at length indicated mild interest in acquiring a quart of milk. Vermont being Vermont, this did not produce warmth or much conversation, but from then on the level of hostility plainly decreased.

Buffering is a necessary courtesy in many societies. Only in high-pressure environments does it tend to disappear—at great cost in bad tempers, ulcers, and heart trouble. If we think in proster terms, it is easy to see an explanation.

Where people routinely work together and regularly carry on activities via well-established prosters, we likely find maximum frequency of interaction with a low rate of active antagonism. Mutually supportive, well-greased prosters tend to hold a group together. The vaunted pregame speeches of football coaches may have value, but bets may more safely be placed on the team that by practice has built the mutually supportive prosters that *are* teamwork. Man was once a hunting animal; just such kind of effort meant triumph, food, injury escaped, and survival.

Our main problem in effecting change, in ourselves or others, too often begins with greatly underestimating the resistance involved, as well as misjudging its nature. Picture a small bit of dead leaf caught on a large spider's web, with our assignment being to move it to a new location an inch away. The effort to do so distorts the entire web. The bit of leaf is held by a network, not by a strand. Similarly, the biases that lead us to select and use a particular proster and program compose an intricate, complex set of interactive factors. It seems simple enough to say, "Don't use that program, use this one" (don't leave the cap off the toothpaste, screw it back on), but the injunction or request or threat does very little to change the set of biases. When we wish to change our own habit, whether smoking, overeating, overusing "that's right" or yah," losing our glasses, or tailgating the car ahead, we find the same difficulty. We think in terms of outcome desired, but not of changing the biases. But the biases select the program, and before we know it, it has been put into effect.

To change a habit, ideally we need two steps. The first is to set up an automatic abortion—something that will interrupt the normal automatic switching-in of the well-established program without attention. If you really want to stop smoking, put a few rubber bands around your pack of cigarettes so they have to be untangled to permit taking one out. The bands will produce anger as they cause abortion of your usual programs, but they will force the matter to your attention, giving you a chance to resist. Second, begin your effort as you begin some major shift of usual environment; for example, being sick in bed or in a hospital, or on a trip or vacation. The more the usual biases are altered, the less the web holds onto the programs you are trying to change.[1]

To illustrate biasing in terms of human interaction, let's consider Tom and Mary, whose marriage is being weakened by incessant quarrels. Tom, let us say, is an industrial engineer with a new, demanding job. Soon after four o'clock, he rushes for his car and the daily battle for the parking-lot exits—400 cars, three exits. On the rest of the thirty mile trip home, Tom can expect to run into more traffic jams, each an abortion of his overall program—driving home —and productive of anger. By the time he reaches his house, Tom is tired and frustrated. Programmatically, he drives into the garage area behind the house, but fairly often one of their children may have left a bike or toy in the way. Angrily, Tom gets out, removes it, rehearses a reproach for his wife, and gets the car down the last few feet of driveway. Now he enters the kitchen door, where Mary— trapped in the house most days because Tom needs their only car to get to work—is preparing dinner, feeding the baby, watching the older children, and fixing a meal for the dog and cat. There is no buffer; suddenly Tom is in the kitchen, perhaps with a complaint. Tom has expectation or plan prosters, based on *his* childhood, where the father played the role of breadwinner to the hilt and the mother made a ceremony of the head of the household returning. Mary has expectation prosters, too. She worked before the first child came, and plans to again. In *her* childhood home, the females were fussed over, flattered, and frequently kissed.

The biases thus are all set like fuses. Only a spark is needed to set off the explosion.

If they go to a marriage counselor, they won't talk about biases. Mary will complain that Tom is too tense, too demanding, unappreciative. Tom will protest that Mary doesn't respond to his needs, doesn't realize how hard he works, doesn't show affection. But suppose they did first reduce the problems to proster and bias terms?

We might find a bit later that Tom sees there is no real reason to rush home. He goes to the plant snack bar to relax and have a bite. When he gets in his car the lot is now nearly empty, and there is no battle for the gate. He still meets jams on the road home, but since he is trying to arrive a little later, the abortion effect is reduced. Instead of coming directly home, he may stop in a park or elsewhere along the route and indulge his hobby of photography for a few minutes. He parks in front of his house, and rings the bell twice to warn Mary of his return, giving her a ten-second buffer to "shift gears." She has fed the baby and the pets, got supper well under way, and now goes into the front room to greet Tom. Warm kiss. Words of affection. Tom takes the children. Curtain.

The problem and solution have been set forth simplistically, of course. Yet even this fable may suggest that when we view behaviors in proster terms, and see the need to change biases rather than attempt to affect behavior directly, we acquire an enormously more practical view of what is happening, and how the stresses can be relieved and necessary changes brought about.

We agonize over crime, and some politicians find that a call for harsher punishments wins some popular approval. But take a look at the man just released from prison after a long sentence. Usually no new prosters of use "outside" have been built during these years. With a few dollars in the pocket of his cheap suit, he is suddenly thrown back into pretty much the same environment he came from, into the complete net of biases that produced the previous criminal acts—and he still has the same prosters and expectation prosters. The result is almost inevitable: the old biases acting on the old prosters produce the same selection, and often the criminal is back at previous pursuits before two days have elapsed. Recidivism for most classes of older criminals approaches 100 percent!

An individual can put into effect only those prosters that have been established. The choice of specific program can only be made from programs available. We cannot play the flute or juggle or make a fine speech because someone orders us to or threatens punishment if we don't, if suitable prosters do not exist. It is no easier for the bank robber to become a shipping clerk than vice versa. One has to learn a role by acquiring programs, grouped in prosters, that permit selecting appropriate actions. As a nation we seem to make little headway against crime because we think in terms of wickedness and punishment. A shift to prosters and biasing might produce startlingly better results.

My object here is to suggest that, if Proster Theory has validity, it can open doors for new approaches to a lot of previously resistant problems. The whole field of neurosis, the maladjustment that produces so much human agony, seems to cry for examination in proster terms—in the severe neurotic, the precisely repeated program (producing futile or negative results, to the embarrassment of all believers in reinforcement) could hardly be more apparent. For any large organization, including the military and police forces, seeking to obtain certain behaviors and appropriate, need-sensitive selection of behaviors in varying circumstances, the proster approach appears to offer possibilities of sharp improvement in methods. The same may hold true for developing the highly skilled people we plainly need in so many areas of activity.

Possibly it is well to reiterate that applying the proster view to behavior is far removed from molding or manipulating approaches that attempt to suppress or deny individual differences. Proster Theory starts from the opposite pole: that no two brains are alike, no two have proster content and organization even closely similar. When we deal with humans with full recognition of differences, we may well have greater success in achieving good relations and more positive, productive, mutually advantageous results.

In sum, we must approach understanding of human behavior by being aware that people do or do not have specific programs available; that they can use only those they have; that selection from among those available will reflect total biasing; and that in-body and ambient factors, and perhaps more built-in influences than we realize, always add further complexity.

We do not simplify human behavior by taking the proster viewpoint; rather we become better prepared to understand and deal with the complexity.

CHAPTER 24

Where Do We Go from Here to Survive?

SOME MUSEUM should acquire me one of these days for later exhibition in a glass case. The plaque beneath it will identify me as one of the last members of the last generation of our society to which "grandfather wisdom" was of appreciable use.

By that term I mean knowledge or rule of practical import that was often handed by grandparent to parent to child, or, in short, idea or information that would stay reasonably valid and in effect over a span of thirty or so years.

Today, even parental wisdom may have an antique flavor. If my grown children do me the occasional courtesy of inviting some counsel (thought of, possibly, as "humoring the old folks"), I must remind myself to be cautious about drawing on *my* experience, unless quite recent. One startling aspect of present times is that the middle-aged routinely pick up from youth a variety of new behaviors—not handed down but handed up—that include gayer and less "proper" clothing, freer spending, and franker sexuality, not to mention accepting and using, even in literature, gobs of new language. Handing along, handing down, still continues, to be sure, but the old certainty that "this is the right way" now is often absent for both the donor and the recipient.

To comment on the rapidity of change is to commit a cliché; but we less commonly note the demise of grandfather wisdom. Mankind has been around for quite a period, and handed-down grandfather wisdom plainly has had a great deal to do with achieving survival. Of all creatures on earth, only man acquired the ability to accumulate and culturally transmit complex bodies of knowledge and belief across two generations—a competence far beyond the limits of parent instructing offspring.

For all but the last tiny fraction of man's history, survival favored those humans who handed along the culture with extremely little change. Age and wisdom went arm in arm: the elders made the group's decisions; the sage was one who had survived longer than most. Tradition, religion, superstition combined as effective preservatives. Man could accommodate much change, under pressure of necessity, and we can assume curiosity grew with increasing alertness and intelligence; but change came slowly and almost exclusively with respect to new events, new things. Most that was new was rejected. Some small part, accepted, was added to the old, and in time became fully part of the traditional culture, equally protected and passed on intact.

It is one thing to add, quite another to replace.

The weight of evidence strongly suggests that once we have constructed prosters in the brain, they remain there for a lifetime. Pavlov himself found that "extinction" did not extinguish, and a thousand experiments since have shown that learning stays, even if apparently unused, for decades. The brain then may be regarded as an accumulating device, and culture as a brain squared, so to speak: an accumulating device for accumulating devices. So the brain has been used through all the generations of mankind; and so it is still used in those present societies—we call them "backward"—that have not yet acquired much skill with that master tool, scientific method.

Now we must tell this adult human brain that has done so well by accumulating to do just the opposite: to de-accumulate, scrap, discard, edit out, replace.

Again and again we find that grandfather wisdom, and even knowledge and concepts we acquired within our own adulthood, do not fit the world we presently live in. We think of evolution as requiring eons to take effect, and then read that a research team has forced "flu germs" to evolve in a few years in the laboratory. Or we learn that a nuclear breeder reactor, after burning its fuel for a period, will have *more* fuel than it started with. For a lifetime, a fast typist was one who could hammer out seventy words a minute, and now we are confronted with a computer's printer that can spew out 1,200 typed *lines* in that time. We must shake our intellect as a wet dog shakes his coat, and send old notions flying.

Even more upsetting are the changes that have successively become manifest in terms of interactions. The latest far-off war is thrust into our living room, the victims' burns black and the wounds gory red. Ethnic groups once seen as docile now picket and protest. Youths at college, previously considered the ultimate of the privileged, seem unappreciative; the once-timid teacher's union shuts down the schools and defies the courts; the house whose doors stayed unlocked for years now must bolt and bar against the burglar, who may be a neighborhood youth seeking kicks or cash for drugs.

The human brain was not built to cope with his kind of continual, crashing, shattering change.

In *The Emergence of Man* Professor John E. Pfeiffer notes that in societies that did not change appreciably over many centuries, survival favored rapid, once-and-for-all learning. But no longer:

> The emphasis must be increasingly on flexibility. The mark of the new evolution which sweeps us along is that unlearning and learning anew have already become as important to survival as learning used to be. What man knows is far less important than his capacity for modifying or discarding what he thinks he knows. . . . The question for the future is whether the built-in flexibility, one of the most distinctive marks of being human, is great enough to permit the erasing if necessary of information learned early—whether in a sense we can be taught to forget as effectively as we remember.[1]

To replace, we must not only add the new proster (which requires time), but also shift and reorganize a great network of biases that have long selected programs from old prosters. Learning takes time and energy. Unlearning, replacing, letting go what used to work—this is far more difficult and demanding in every sense. We see the problem illustrated, in a way, when some infuriatingly stubborn computer cannot let loose of the conviction that we owe for a patchwork bedspread, a nine-minute phone call to Carefree, Arizona, or 40,000 empty oil drums, that respectively we returned, didn't make, or never heard of. Compared in complexity to our brain, remember, the computer is a simple toy.

In proster terms, change upsets **and** perhaps deeply disturbs us because it aborts programs that used to serve well, and forces in adults the continual revision of the world-as-perceived that has always been normal in children. Becoming an adult has always meant acquiring a foundation-set of understandings that we could rely on to a reasonable degree without dependence on others; and to have this foundation shrink, to be in that sense thrust back into childhood, may prove intolerable. The effect is pervasive, though subtle. We feel that the world is out of joint, that it may be futile to try to set it right.

Hebb and others have pointed out that adults are not really less emotional than children, but more.[2] We feel stronger emotions, much longer. With experience, however, we acquire prosters for handling —and to a large degree in our society, "corking up"—the more visible emotions. And as we develop skill in operating within our individual worlds, we tend to build a shell around ourselves, like a spore, and live within this armor, avoiding activities or places where it might be penetrated.

"I do not want to get involved" serves as a watchword for many, perhaps to a greater extent than the individual realizes. We appear to have far fewer people today than forty years ago who hold strong, durable commitments in politics, patriotism, religious affiliations and theology, community affairs, or even marriage, family unity, and common morality. Employers complain that their employees don't care, steal, quit and move for trivial reasons—especially the younger ones. Union leaders voice much the same complaint about their membership, to whom the old battle cries may seem fusty ancient history. Suburban homeowners typically behave as if their deed bought not only land and house but a guarantee of immunity—on "our block"—from all social problems and change to meet them. Corruption sweeps through police forces, and investigations show some defenders of law and order engage not only in bribe-taking but also theft, burglary, and drug pushing. Commitment fails to keep district attorneys and legislators from indictment and conviction, and when boards of education meet to discuss how children can be taught more respect for authority, they must bear in mind that the nation's most publicized wrongdoers have populated the White House itself. It seems as if our world is coming apart at the seams like an overloaded inflated boat in rough waters. The effect is stunning, stupefying.

But before we become too pessimistic, and wring our hands raw in despair, consider once again the proposition that we can only use those programs we have established and have available. What appears to be apathy or withdrawal or rejection may be no more than a symptom of lack of programs appropriate to these biases. To behave in our usual ways doesn't work, but we lack substitutes—or we fail to recognize new programs in that light.

If we look to our young adult generation, we seem at first to find even more grounds for discouragement. In political action, civil rights, environmental protection, peace, educational reform, quality of life, and other key issue areas, the involvement of young people appears spasmodic and short-lived. The enthusiasm, even the violence, of a few years ago seems to have burned out, leaving scarcely a trace. The communes, religious movements, back-to-nature groups, encounter and mysticism devotees all seem to move toward withdrawal rather than struggle with evident problems.

But perhaps we do not really see what is going on. All these dismal symptoms of collapse and rotting institutions, distressing and even revolting as they may be, can also be viewed as part of the erasing process Pfeiffer refers to. Certainly older citizens manage to detect in the younger a letting go of old rigidities not long ago regarded as good manners, proper behavior, correct relationships, respectability, and prescribed ethics. Most of the weddings I have attended lately, for example, have been of couples who have been living together fairly openly. It seems apparent they married legally not to be free to enjoy sexual activity, but for less carnal reasons—a reordering that is not automatically a loss, it would seem, however much it may outrage some defenders of old institutions. Youngsters have decided in considerable numbers that rushing off to college is an idea they can let go. The film *American Graffiti* reminds us how much the obsession with "wheels" has dimmed, even before gasoline pinches laid on a cold restraining hand.

Letting go, erasing, unlearning can be a process harder to see than the decay of aged institutions—but one more cheering.

We may gain perspective when we remind ourselves of the three-in-one structure of the human brain. Our oldest brain fiercely clings to distant eras of existence on a primitive level; our middle one, though far more intricate, is tied to emotional expression rather than complex ideas and verbalization, and it too is past-oriented. Only the newest brain has the flexibility to cope reasonably willingly with new matters.

But it does so, we must always remember, by utilizing new combinations or applications of what it already has stored—much as a mechanic, faced with a kind of fastener he has never encountered before, rummages in his tool box for something there he can use to remove it. The cortex first seeks solutions by using previous learning, not by unlearning.

And the new brain, as we have seen, is a nervous prima donna, able and willing to perform at best only when conditions seem just right. Under threat, our brains downshift. The need to let go, to unlearn, to replace—frequently, suddenly, violently—can itself be seen as threat.

Change, flooding in constantly, demanding unlearning and replacement, produces fear. Fear brings downshifting, and so less ability to cope cerebrally with change. This seems to be the circular problem that underlies the anxieties of our times.

It can scarcely be dismissed as either a light or temporary problem. Possibly we may not survive as a species too much longer, unless we find ways to relieve it. With a magnificent cortex able to change the world at breakneck speed, but a lack of offsetting apparatus to accept and control our own human works, we may end up too much out of balance to exist.

The key to survival, I suggest, lies in gaining new and insightful understanding of the human brain, its history, its nature, and its functioning.

To break the circle of fear producing downshifting, we need to remember that the antidote to downshifting, to inability to use the enormous latent power of the human brain, is confidence. We produce only a sprinkling of confident people who do not readily downshift in the face of change and the abortion of old programs, who take for granted both the continuing need and their ability to unlearn and replace. Perhaps our newest adults, in more and more resisting empty credentialing and acceptance of discredited authorities, have made more progress than seems evident.

The biggest block to increasing the proportion of confident people is of course our long-outmoded educational system, and in particular our schools. While our need for confident flexibility grows acute, they still foster rigidity, the right answer, "permanent" learning attested by credentials, learning as preparation, learning as something forced on a victim—learning divorced from life, reality, individuality, and human needs. Happy exceptions increase, but they are still very few.

But not only in child rearing and education but throughout our society, we seem in urgent need of entering the skull, to acquire fresh understanding of the brain that makes us human and of why it today must cope with unprecedented demands. To suppress rather than increasingly use its stupendous power is to carry brinksmanship to a new extreme.

Working from many directions, investigators of the brain have steadily converged toward a unified conception, a body of knowledge and theory that has become mutually supportive. It appears to offer a foundation with a solidity we fail to find in the many nonbrain schools of psychology, psychiatry, and the social sciences at present. On it we can build comprehensive theory of how the brain works that may permit early and broad application.

It can be encouraging to reflect that electricity and its genius stepchild, electronics, serve us at every turn; yet roughly a century ago even the basics of electricity were scarcely understood, and electronics unheard of, by most people. The impact of brain theory could prove even more pervasive, its solidification and broad application a landmark in the history of man as significant as our coming down from the trees to walk erect upon the earth.

NOTES

CHAPTER 1

1. Ernest Gardner, *Fundamentals of Neurology*, 5th edition (Philadelphia: W. B. Saunders, 1968), p. 175.

2. For example, *Educational Psychology, A Contemporary View* (Del Mar, California: CRM Books, 1973) has no entry under "brain," "central nervous system," or "nervous system." Though this handsome, elaborate 457-page book lists more than sixty prominent "contributing consultants," most of them with impressive academic credentials and associated with a wide variety of university or other institutions, brain is almost totally ignored throughout. The introduction is addressed to the "future teacher."

3. Of some 150 articles that appeared during 1973 in *The Education Digest*, from a wide range of sources, not a single one had "brain" or an equivalent term in the title. This respected publication reflects broad coverage of current educational literature.

4. A typical comment on this point is by Chester A. Lawson of Michigan State University: "It is probably no exaggeration to say that the average teacher makes little or no use of learning theory in his day-to-day classroom activities. This may be due to his ignorance of theories of learning, or it may be due to the irrelevance of current learning theories to the problems of human learning." Chester A. Lawson, *Brain Mechanisms and Human Learning* (Boston: Houghton Mifflin, 1967), p. xi.

5. Under the general heading of "behavior modification," similar control efforts have been experimented with in prison, mental hospital, and other confinement settings, usually under the gloss of "benefiting the inmates." Some of these have been cruel, arrogant, irresponsible experimentation with human beings, literally beyond belief. As instances have been exposed (some by the American Civil Liberties Union) such abuses have been slowed, but probably not stopped.

6. Bergen Richard Bugelski, *The Psychology of Learning Applied to Teaching*, 2d edition (Indianapolis: Bobbs-Merrill, 1971), p. vii.

7. Donald M. Medley and Harold E. Mitzel, "The Scientific Study of Teacher Behavior," in *Theory and Research in Teaching*, ed. Arno A. Bellack (New York: Teachers College Press, Columbia University, 1963), p. 82.

8. Ernest R. Hilgard, ed., *Theories of Learning and Instruction*, Sixty-third Yearbook of the National Society for the Study of Education, part 1 (Chicago: University of Chicago Press, 1964), p. 171.

9. Jerome S. Bruner, *Toward A Theory of Instruction* (New York: W. W. Norton, 1968), pp. 31, 37.

10. U. S. Office of Education estimate for 1972–73. See *American Education*, October 1972, pp. 4–7.

CHAPTER 2

1. A. R. Luria, "The Functional Organization of the Brain," *Scientific American*, March 1970, p. 66. See also A. R. Luria, *The Working Brain* (New York: Basic Books, 1974), p. 79, for reference to programs.

2. Karl H. Pribram, "Neurological Notes on the Art of Educating," in *Theories of Learning and Instruction*, Sixty-third Yearbook of the National Society for the Study of Education: 1964, p. 102. See also George A. Miller, E. Galenter, and Karl H. Pribram, *Plans and the Structure of Behavior* (New York: Henry Holt, 1960).

3. The brilliantly original and practical Dr. Omar Khayyam Moore of the University of Pittsburgh has suggested a test of any learning theory: can it account for the things we know human beings do learn?

4. See, for example, the article by Peter Stoler in *Time*, January 14, 1974, pp. 50–59, which surveys some major areas of current research.

5. Luria, *The Working Brain*, p. 41.

CHAPTER 3

1. David Pilbeam, "An Idea We Could Live Without," *Discovery 7*, Spring 1972, pp. 65–66.

2. Arthur W. Staats, *Learning, Language and Cognition* (New York: Holt, Rinehart and Winston, 1968), p. 87.

3. Howard Rachlin, *Introduction to Modern Behaviorism* (San Francisco: W. H. Freeman, 1970), p. 59.

4. René Dubos, *So Human an Animal* (New York: Charles Scribner's Sons, 1968), p. 216.

5. Dr. Carl Rogers, former president of the American Psychological Association, has commented: "I guess psychologists are about the most defensive professional people around today. We have this terrific fear of looking unscientific. A terrific fear of spinning out wild theories to see how they sound, and a fear of trying them out. We think we must do everything from a *known* base with *known* instruments. Actually, this is *not* the way in which creative scientists, even in the hard sciences, operate." Mary Harrington Hall, "A Conversation with Carl Rogers," in *Readings in Psychology Today*, 2d edition (Del Mar, Calif.: CRM Books, 1972), p. 449.

6. J. McVicker Hunt, "The Psychological Basis for Using Pre-School Enrichment as an Antidote for Cultural Deprivation," in *Children: Readings in Behavior and Development*, ed. by Ellis D. Evans (New York: Holt, Rinehart and Winston, 1968), p. 485.

7. Herbert A. Thelen, *Education and the Human Quest* (New York: Harper & Row, 1960), p. 2.

8. The unhappiness of psychologists with conventional American psychology has produced a growing literature. For a documented and often devastating review, see Benjamin M. Braginsky and Dorothea D. Braginsky, *Mainstream Psychology* (New York: Holt, Rinehart and Winston, 1974). Early in the book the collaborators remark: "As psychologists, we are committed to the survival of psychology as a viable system for truth-seeking. . . . So long as its foundations are myths, absurdities, and pretensions, its demise is inevitable" (p. 4). In recommending redirection, the authors do not venture far into the field of brain. The word does not appear in the table of contents or index, and only passing references suggest that there is anything inside the human skull.

CHAPTER 4

1. In 1967 a jawbone fragment, considered to be evidence of *Australopithecus*, was found in the Lake Rudolph region of Kenya by a team headed by Professor Bryan Patterson. It later was dated at 5.5 million years old. In the same area, Richard Leakey found a fragmented, large-brained skull dated as at least 2.6 million years old, pushing the age of this premodern development back about a million years. The geology of the region favors relatively accurate datings. Apparently *Australopithecus* and more modern forms lived at the same time. (See *New York Times*, November 10, 1972.)

2. For one of the soundest and clearest discussions of the topic, see John E. Pfeiffer, *The Emergence of Man* (New York: Harper & Row, 1969). Pfeiffer is a professor of anthropology at Rutgers University.

3. If curriculum is taken as a guide, almost every high school teaches evolutionary theory, and the subject gets some attention at lower levels as well. In practice, however, my experience has been that even top-ranked seniors have trouble recalling ever having studied evolution, and have only the haziest notion of the main tenets. Our educational system appears to regard the learning of, say, Euclidean geometry as worth far more effort than achieving some understanding of the principles that underlie our existence and survival as humans. Or it may be that evolution remains a topic still capable of arousing parental ire on religious grounds, and so gets at best nominal attention in most schools.

4. See H. B. D. Kettlewell, "Darwin's Missing Evidence," *Scientific American*, March 1959, p. 48.

5. Dean E. Wooldridge, *The Machinery of the Brain* (New York: McGraw-Hill, 1963), p. 81.

6. Lionel Tiger and Robin Fox, *The Imperial Animal* (New York: Holt, Rinehart and Winston, 1971), p. 61.

7. By analysis of the oxygen in ice taken from bore holes in the Greenland ice sheet, climate changes for 125,000 years back have been closely estimated. An exceptionally abrupt "little ice age" occurred between 90,000 and 89,000 years ago. For a report on an international conference on the subject, see the *New York Times*, February 5, 1972. Climate oscillation may have begun two million or more years ago. See Pfeiffer, *Emergence of Man*, p. 101.

8. For a discussion of brain sizes, see Pfeiffer, *Emergence of Man*, p. 105.

CHAPTER 5

1. James P. Chaplin, *Dictionary of Psychology* (New York: Dell, 1968), p. 303.

2. Newell C. Kephart, *The Slow Learner in the Classroom* (Columbus, Ohio: Charles E. Merrill, 1960), p. 67.

3. Donald O. Hebb, "Drive and the C. N. S. (Conceptual [*sic*] Nervous System)," *Psychological Review* 62 (1955): 243–254. The paper was a presidential address to the American Psychological Association.

4. One does not have to go back more than a few decades in the literature to find estimates of the number of neurons as low as one or two billion. Today, thirty billion would be viewed as quite a modest figure by some investigators, but even this estimate is so staggering that larger ones would seem almost pointless for most purposes—it is hard to conceive of functions that could not be performed, with much redundancy, by this quantity of richly interconnected neuron units.

CHAPTER 6

1. For a discussion of adaptations required in creatures emerging from life solely in water, see Everett C. Olson, *The Evolution of Life* (New York: New American Library, 1965), p. 169.

2. "The brain is no mere decorative flower at the top of the evolutionary tree. Even if we never used it for thinking, we would still need it, merely to keep us alive. It is first of all the body's organ of adjustment . . . it activates, co-ordinates, and regulates the body in all . . . its relationships to the environment without. The cell's metabolism, the functioning of organs and systems are all watched over by the brain." Benjamin F. Miller and Ruth Goode, *Man and His Body* (New York: Simon and Schuster, 1960), p. 273. This lucid work offers a perceptive introduction to the human organism. Part 5, "The Great Integrator," deals with the nervous system.

3. The lack of interest in evolutionary approach is evidenced in the literature. For example, the widely used and respected text by Robert M. W. Travers, *Essentials of Learning*, 3rd edition (New York: Macmillan, 1972), has no "evolution" entry in the index. Nor does the equally outstanding work by Ernest R. Hilgard and Gordon H. Bower, *Theories of Learning*, 3rd edition (New York: Appleton-Century-Crofts, 1966). Both are exhaustive surveys, notable also in that each has an entire chapter on the nervous system.

4. See Olson, *Evolution of Life*, p. 45.

5. For a clear and detailed discussion, see C. U. M. Smith, *The Brain* (New York: G. P. Putnam's Sons, 1970), chapter 10, "The Evolution of Vertebrate Brains," pp. 195–213.

6. Ibid., p. 209.

CHAPTER 7

1. Niko Tinbergen, *The Herring Gull's World* (New York: Basic Books, 1960). See particularly the illustrations facing pp. 192–193. The same author's *Social Behavior in Animals* (London: Methuen, 1953) deals with a number of species. For a virtual encyclopedia of behaviors in popular but authoritative presentation, see the superbly illustrated *Fascinating World of Animals* (Pleasantville, N. Y.: The Reader's Digest Association, 1971).

2. Recognition of pattern can also be built-in. A well-known example from ethological sources is the experimental towing of a dummy bird with a wing-span and body extending from it. When towed with the body in front of the wings, a gooselike silhouette, chicks on the ground showed no alarm. Reversed and towed with wings in front, like a hawk, the chicks froze at once—even though they had never seen a hawk. For a convenient reference, see Roger Tory Peterson, *The Birds*, Life Nature Library (New York: Time, 1963), p. 123.

3. Beginning in the 1950s, as electronic devices proliferated, a number of such robots were created experimentally by W. R. Ashby, W. Grey Walter, J. A. Deutsch, and others. They proved capable of behaviors which could be called "foraging for food," "learning a maze," and other designed-in tasks or programs—even "coming home when tired."

4. Pribram has expressed a similar view succinctly: "Freedom is not anarchy. Real freedom is intelligent, knowledgeable choice and rises out of order when order achieves sufficient complexity." See Karl H. Pribram, "Neurological Notes on the Art of Educating," in *Theories of Learning and Instruction*, ed. Ernest R. Hilgard, Sixty-third Yearbook of the National Society for the Study of Education, part 1 (Chicago: University of Chicago Press, 1964), p. 108.

5. For discussions of the brain's two-sidedness, see Robert W. Sperry, "The Great Cerebral Commissure," *Scientific American*, January 1964, p. 42; and Michael S. Gazzaniga, "The Split Brain in Man," *Scientific American*, August 1967, p. 24. A number of cases in which the corpus callosum, the bridge between the two hemispheres, has been cut for medical reasons have thrown much light on the assignments the two sides have in humans, in whom the need to deal with words requires allotting a large amount of brain resources to this characteristically human activity. A split brain, of course, should not be regarded as directly reflecting the operation of the two sides in a normal brain—the differences likely become exaggerated to at least some degree. The size of the corpus callosum suggests a great deal of exchange and mutual influencing in the intact brain.

6. References to the case appear throughout the literature. It occurred in 1848. See Dean E. Wooldridge, *The Machinery of the Brain* (New York: McGraw-Hill, 1963), p. 146, for a good account. For a more modern report on a similar case, see J. Lawrence Pool, *Your Brain and Nerves* (New York: Charles Scribner's Sons, 1973), pp. 50–51. Dr. Pool is an eminent neurosurgeon, and professor at Columbia University.

7. A. R. Luria, "The Functional Organization of the Brain," *Scientific American*, March 1970, p. 66.

CHAPTER 8

1. Emotions, long ago seen as some form of demon in possession, have in our century been regarded as "an awareness, a distinctive conscious process that is quite separate from intellectual processes." The words are those of the distinguished and innovative psychologist Donald Hebb. He continues: "This notion has led to a good deal of confusion, for it has gradually become clear that no such distinct kind of awareness exists." Though Hebb reported "a surprising unanimity of psychological opinion" on this point a quarter-century ago, the notion continues to be a common belief, and practically an article of basic faith among educators, who often refer to "affective" and "cognitive" areas as though they were separate, unconnected, and even opposite. Donald O. Hebb, *The Organization of Behavior* (New York: John Wiley, 1949), p. 147.

2. Nigel Calder, *The Mind of Man* (New York: Viking Press, 1970), p. 58.

3. Pribram notes of "behavioral expressions of emotional feelings" that they "signify the interests" of the organism by serving as signals in a social environment. Pribram, *Languages of the Brain* (Englewood Cliffs, N.J.: Prentice-Hall, 1971), p. 213.

4. Calder, *The Mind of Man*, chapter 5, "An Inward Spaceflight," pp. 80–95. It includes discussion of the remarkable work of Dr. Neal Miller, who persistently clung to an "absurd" line of research until, at an international assembly of psychologists in 1969, he shattered the old "autonomous" concept once and for all.

5. See José M. R. Delgado, *Physical Control of the Mind* (New York: Harper & Row, 1969) for a discussion of this technique and findings from its use.

CHAPTER 9

1. See C. U. M. Smith, *The Brain*, p. 118. The range in humans is probably somewhat less, within these extremes.

2. Hierarchical organization of the brain as a fundamental principle of its operation is widely accepted among leading neuroscientists, and referred to in the literature in many connections. The concept—if not necessarily my explanations here—constitutes a cornerstone of present brain understanding. The old notion of conscious and unconscious, insofar as it suggests a simple division into two parts, has little present usefulness.

CHAPTER 10

1. For an accurate report on Moore's astonishing achievements using a "responsive environment" technique he and associates developed, see Maya Pines, *Revolution in Learning* (New York: Harper & Row, 1967), chapter 5, "The Talking Typewriter." Further work in Pittsburgh and Chicago has sustained the effectiveness of Moore's approaches, but the findings appear to be so uncomfortable for most conventional educators that the work of Moore has

won only occasional, usually grudging references rather than excited attention.

2. C. U. M. Smith, *The Brain* (New York: G. P. Putnam's Sons, 1970), p. 141. Alfred North Whitehead, in *The Aims of Education* (New York: New American Library, 1964), refers to "that stream of events that pours through" a child's life and *is* his life (p. 14).

3. Many classroom teachers seem sincerely convinced that they "individualize" in handling their students, but study after study fails to produce evidence that they in fact do. Rather, observers find teachers in classrooms behave in remarkably similar "group" ways. See John I. Goodlad, M. Frances Klein, and associates, *Looking Behind the Classroom Door* (Worthington, Ohio: Charles A. Jones, 1974); and Raymond S. Adams and Bruce J. Biddle, *Realities of Teaching* (New York: Holt, Rinehart and Winston, 1970). The conventional classroom, as a setting, appears to coerce teachers into a narrow pattern. For an analysis of the classroom structure and its effects, see Leslie A. Hart, *The Classroom Disaster* (New York: Teachers College Press, Columbia University, 1969).

CHAPTER 11

1. See Peter Nathan, *The Nervous System* (Philadelphia: J. B. Lippincott, 1969), p. 158; see also discussion, p. 258.

2. See Steven Rose, *The Conscious Brain* (New York: Alfred A. Knopf, 1973), p. 46.

3. For a brief summary of one famous sensory deprivation experiment, see Donald O. Hebb, *Textbook of Psychology*, 3rd edition (Philadelphia: W. B. Saunders, 1972), pp. 212–13. He remarks of some of the students who underwent the experience that their "very identity had begun to disintegrate." For a detailed discussion, see Woodburn Heron, "The Pathology of Boredom," *Scientific American*, January 1957, p. 52.

4. Peter Nathan, *The Nervous System*, p. 157.

5. Desmond Morris, *The Human Zoo* (New York: McGraw-Hill, 1969), p. 184.

CHAPTER 12

1. Various bits of evidence seem to suggest that identification of a color or aural tone rests predominantly on comparison of just *two* key factors, and we may speculate that this two-element keying is a basic characteristic of brain function, serving to simplify and speed handling of very complex inputs. For rough analogy, our use of a first and last name to identify individuals provides an easy, fast way of sorting out, at least tentatively, a particular individual from among millions. See Edwin H. Land, "Experiments in Color Vision," *Scientific American*, May 1959, p. 84.

2. The brilliant work of David H. Hubel and Torsten N. Wiesel, and the earlier findings of Stephen W. Kuffler, have shown that the retina and visual-processing areas in the brain deal with bits and pieces of information—edges, contrasts, angle of orientation, direction of movement, or other change— which the brain somehow assembles, in effect, into the picture or image we

see. For a discussion in some detail of these investigations, see David H. Hubel, "The Visual Cortex of the Brain," *Scientific American*, November 1963, p. 54.

3. The code is basically the same for all senses. Vision is vision because the code is received and processed by certain neuron networks that interpret any input as visual. A blow on the eye makes us "see stars" because it fired impulses over visual tracts.

4. This idea that nerve channels bring in codes that we must learn to recognize before perception occurs startles many people, I have found in lecturing on Proster Theory to various groups. Yet as long ago as 1867, Hermann von Helmholtz was telling large audiences: "All that we apprehend of the external world is brought to our consciousness by means of certain changes which are produced in our organs of sense by external impressions, and transmitted to the brain by the nerves. It is in the brain that these impressions first become conscious sensations, and are combined so as to produce our conceptions of surrounding objects." He strongly supported what was then called the Empirical Theory of Vision, which held that "None of our sensations give us anything more than 'signs' . . . we can only learn how to interpret these signs by means of experience and practice." See *Helmholtz on Perception, ed.* Richard M. Warren and Roslyn P. Warren (New York: John Wiley, 1968) p. 82 and p. 110. Helmholtz, surely one of the greatest scientific intellects of all time, astonishingly accurate in his main understandings, suffered the vigorous antagonism of most of his contemporaries who were laying the foundations of the new science of psychology.

5. See Jean Piaget and Barbel Inhelder, *Mental Imagery in the Child*, translated by P. A. Chilton (New York: Basic Books, 1971), p. 355.

6. Luria states explicitly: "Perception . . . is an active process which includes the search for the most important elements of information, their comparison with each other, the creation of a hypothesis concerning the meaning of the information as a whole, and the verification of this hypothesis by comparing it with the original features of the object perceived. The more complex the object perceived, and the less familiar it is, the more detailed this perceptual activity will be." A. R. Luria, *The Working Brain* (New York: Basic Books, 1974), p. 240.

7. Karl H. Pribram, "Neurological Notes on the Art of Educating," in *Theories of Learning and Instruction*, ed. Ernest R. Hilgard, Sixty-third Yearbook of the National Society for the Study of Education, part 1 (Chicago: University of Chicago Press, 1964), p. 89.

8. Mary A. B. Brazier, "The Analysis of Brain Waves," *Scientific American*, June 1962, p. 150.

CHAPTER 13

1. For a review of receptors in lucid terms, see Peter Nathan, *The Nervous System* (Philadelphia: J. B. Lippincott, 1969), chapters 1–7.

2. Donald G. Fink, in *Computers and the Human Mind* (Garden City, N. Y.: Doubleday, 1966), p. 183, notes an estimate that sense organs generate at least 100 million impulses per second, every second of "our waking lives." However accurate the figure, the input must clearly be on a stupendous scale.

CHAPTER 14

1. The author freely and gratefully acknowledges a great debt to the literature of several disciplines drawn on to formulate Proster Theory. Giving such a name to a synthesis may be regarded by some as presumptuous. I would submit, however, that the economical and clear new language, the organizing device of the proster, and the integration that results may justify the theory format—particularly if it proves useful and provocative in many practical applications.

2. This ingenious laboratory device, automated in varying degrees, may make life misrable for the incarcerated animal, but usually easier for the behaviorist who doesn't even have to watch—in contrast to the ethologist, who has to go out into the field and spend almost all investigative time watching, usually uncomfortably. It has enabled wrong conclusions to be reached far more efficiently.

3. Paul D. MacLean, "Man and His Animal Brains," *Modern Medicine*, February 3, 1964, p. 96.

4. In the laboratory, caged animals, given a shock from an invisible source (the floor grid), will at once attack another of their own species, or an animal of another species, or even a stuffed toy. See Nathan Azrin, "Pain and Aggression," *Psychology Today*, May 1967, p. 26.

5. *Theory Into Practice*, a periodical published by the College of Education of The Ohio State University, devoted its October 1971 issue to "nonverbal awareness."

6. Paul D. MacLean, "New Findings Relevant to the Evolution of Psychosexual Functions of the Brain," *Journal of Nervous and Mental Disease*, 135 (October 1962): 289.

CHAPTER 15

1. Donald O. Hebb, *Textbook of Psychology* (Philadelphia: W. B. Saunders, 1972), p. 198.

2. Observation of downshifting has of course been common, and at times insightful. For example, Arthur W. Combs and Donald Snygg note in *Individual Behavior* (New York: Harper & Row, 1959) that threat narrows perception to what threatens (p. 389). Notable studies of anxiety in learners have been made by Seymour B. Sarason and associates at Yale University. In *Anxiety in Elementary School Children* (New York: John Wiley, 1960), p. 265, Sarason et al. observe that anxiety is painful and brings "defensive or avoidance reactions." They found that teachers often did not recognize anxiety in children to a useful degree, especially in "bright, motivated" students.

CHAPTER 16

1. Peter Nathan, *The Nervous System* (Philadelphia: J. B. Lippincott, 1969), p. 348.

CHAPTER 17

1. The number of neuromuscular "events" in a single minute of ordinary human speech has been estimated at 10,000 to 15,000. See E. H. Lennenberg, *Biological Foundations of Language*, (New York: John Wiley, 1967), p. 107.

2. Astonishingly, even the two human ears "hear" differently, the right usually being better attuned to speech and the left to music. (Like those of the eyes, the nerve pathways for hearing have a strong crossover to the opposite side of the brain.) See Doreen Kimura, "The Asymmetry of the Human Brain," *Scientific American*, March 1973, p. 70.

3. See Ann James Premack and David Premack, "Teaching Language to an Ape," *Scientific American*, October 1972, p. 92; and Joyce Dudney Fleming, "The State of the Apes" and "The Lucy and Roger Talk Show," *Psychology Today*, January 1974, pp. 31, 49.

4. For reasons now less than apparent, a series of three strikes in succession is called a turkey.

5. The situational influences can also produce quite absurd misunderstanding, especially when the situation is ambiguous or multiple. At dinner with some guests, I asked a college student to please pass the grapes. With final examinations on his mind, he heard my request as a question on whether he would get passing grades, and replied accordingly. Studies with recorded, isolated words, completely nonsituational, show listeners have much difficulty "catching" them, and make many errors. Context is all-important for accuracy.

6. The work of Professor Noam Chomsky of the Massachusetts Institute of Technology has enormously influenced modern linguistics. For a useful brief study of the impact of his ideas, see John Lyons, *Chomsky* (London: Fontana Books (Collins), 1970). The point is made: "One of the most striking facts about language is its 'creativity'—the fact that by the age of five or six children are able to produce and understand an indefinitely large number of utterances that they have not previously encountered" (p. 84). The fact gives behaviorists extreme difficulties in explaining the learning of speech.

7. See Victoria A. Fromkin, "Slips of the Tongue," *Scientific American*, December 1973, p. 110 for a discussion on this point. See also Paul A. Kolers, "Experiments in Reading," *Scientific American*, July 1972, p. 84; and, particularly, the chart of errors, p. 90. Kolers's ingenious experiments show "that a reader proceeds not by perceiving letter by letter or even word by word but rather by generating internal grammatical messages" (p. 90).

8. It should be noted that while great stress is often put on evaluations such as reading scores, the literature on educational testing overflows with doubts as to validity, reliability, accuracy, and importance. Instrumental evaluations and such supposed standards as grade level accordingly should not be taken at face value. See Fred T. Wilhelms, ed., *Evaluation as Feedback and Guide: Yearbook of the Association for Supervision and Curriculum Development, NEA* (Washington: ASCD–NEA, 1967).

9. Many jokes of the purely verbal variety appear to depend on this principle. We are led on a certain path, but then the twist suddenly takes us in an unexpected direction. For example, the critic's remark: "I saw the show under rather distressing circumstances—the curtain was up." Many puns in-

volve the same unexpected retracking: "I have to get new plates for my car. It's so old it needs uppers and lowers."

CHAPTER 18

1. Karl H. Pribram, "The Neurophysiology of Remembering," *Scientific American*, January 1969, p. 75.

2. The technique of holography has developed rapidly in recent years with the availability of lasers, but the theory was put forward in 1949, by Dr. Dennis Gabor, the Nobel Prize winner considered the father of the art. For a technical discussion, see John N. Butters, *Holography and Its Technology* (London: Peter Peregrinus, 1971).

3. See Karl H. Pribram, *Languages of the Brain* (Englewood Cliffs, N. J.: Prentice-Hall, 1971) for an extensive discussion, pp. 145–66.

4. Neal E. Miller, quoted in Daniel P. Kimble, ed., *The Anatomy of Memory* (Palo Alto, California: Science and Behavior Books, 1965), equates the capacity to one thousand books (p. 293).

5. See Ward C. Halstead and William B. Rucker, "Memory: A Molecular Maze," *Psychology Today*, June 1968, p. 38. Reprinted in *Readings in Psychology Today*, 2d edition (Del Mar, California: CRM Books, 1972), pp. 125–30.

6. See Ralph Norman Haber, "How We Remember What We See," *Scientific American*, May 1970, p. 104.

7. For a brief summary on the topic, see Donald O. Hebb, *The Organization of Behavior* (New York: John Wiley and Sons, 1949), p. 177.

CHAPTER 19

1. W. Grey Walter, "The Mechanisms of the Mind," in *From Molecule to Man*, ed. J. Z. Young and Tom Margerison (New York: Crown Publishers, 1969), p. 118.

2. See J. McVicker Hunt, *Intelligence and Experience* (New York: Ronald Press, 1961), p. 57 and chapter 3.

3. See Hunt, *Intelligence and Experience.*

4. See Robert L. Fantz, "The Origin of Form Perception," *Scientific American*, May 1961, p. 66.

5. Referring to the important brain properties of "dispersal and plasticity of function," Walter notes that when points within large areas are electrically stimulated the patient notices nothing and continues reading, talking, or sleeping. No functional change appears. These "silent areas" are all over the brain, and their location varies in different people and even from time to time. The largest single area is in the frontal lobes, where "all sensory signals converge and are processed for action or reflection." See Walter, "The Mechanisms of the Mind," in *From Molecule to Man*, p. 118.

6. For a brief discussion, see Leon Festinger, "Cognitive Dissonance," *Scientific American*, October 1962, p. 93. "If a person knows various things

that are not psychologically consistent with one another, he will, in a variety of ways, try to make them more consistent."

7. Actual, traumatic brain damage can of course occur, due to difficult birth, very poor nutrition, or accidents in the early years. Terms like minimal brain damage and the equivalent are commonly used, however, to mean that there is *no* such known history, and *no* direct, physical evidence of brain injury. Where sharp evidence of trauma is lacking, experience seems a far more plausible explanation, with home and school environments prime suspects. Many outstanding adults exhibited behavior in childhood that today might well earn the label "brain damaged," especially as it suits adult convenience to blame the child for being different or nonconforming.

8. See A. R. Luria, *The Working Brain* (New York: Basic Books, 1974), p. 87.

9. The bettor may neurotically want to lose, which brings us into the further complexities of punishment presumably serving as reward.

10. A prominent psychologist, a professor of psychology at San Francisco State College and author of a text widely used in teacher training, observes: "As a result of our commitment to reward-and-punishment principles in learning we have come to confuse *teaching* with *control*. . . . The history of education is littered with the failures of those who believed that learning is the direct outcome of reward and punishment. Nor have employers, prison officials, military leaders, and others charged with the guidance, instruction, and control of persons placed under their supervision done any better using similar methods." Henry Clay Lindgren, *Educational Psychology in the Classroom,* 4th edition (New York: John Wiley, 1972), p. 166. The furor over teaching machines, designed to implement reinforcement theory, reached a peak a decade ago but rapidly faded as experience grossly failed to produce predicted results. Minor interest in computer-assisted instruction lingers on. Both technologies probably have some usefulness, distorted, however, by efforts to apply a false theory.

CHAPTER 20

1. Jerome Kagan, the well-known professor of developmental psychology at Harvard University, has stated this explicitly: "When we say that a new entity is learned, we mean that an element is connected with a second element that already has been learned. No act, idea, image or word is learned in isolation or ever becomes completely isolated. Every mind consists of nests of interconnected elements that are continually being reorganized with use." Without using the term programs, Dr. Kagan observes that "Practice of a skill has the inevitable consequence of making that skill . . . more likely to operate as one unit, rather than a sequence of separate elements." (*New York Times,* January 12, 1970, p. 72.)

2. The reference is to individual or small groups of neurons. Collectively, the brain has a pulse much as the heart has, and maintains overall levels of activity. Random discharges are against this organized background, something like static in an otherwise well-received radio program.

CHAPTER 21

1. The National Assessment of Educational Progress is a continuing effort to determine what students and young adults know, from whatever sources, by testing a representative sample. Findings are published from time to time. It is conducted by the Educational Commission of the States, based in Denver, Colorado.

2. The range of differences among humans is seldom given full attention or long remembered, it would seem, even by those who give lip service to recognition of differences. For an engrossing review of how greatly and in how many ways individuals differ, see Roger J. Williams, *You Are Extraordinary* (New York: Random House, 1967). Chapter 3 deals with the nervous system.

3. For a notable experiment using animals, whose changes in brain anatomy and chemistry could be directly verified, see Mark R. Rosenzweig, Edward L. Bennett, and Marian Cleeves Diamond, "Brain Changes in Response to Experience," *Scientific American*, February 1972, p. 22.

4. See Caleb Gattegno, *Towards A Visual Culture* (New York: Outerbridge & Dienstfrey, 1969), p. 34.

5. We should note that labels are often essential, as a practical requirement, to get children admitted to such public facilities as exist for the unwanted child. It becomes to the advantage of the parents, the operators of the institution, the social workers involved, and the child—if old enough to realize the issue—to maintain the label. A so-called retarded boy, for example, if found "normal," would likely have to be expelled from the institution and for lack of alternatives might well end up in some kind of prison. Considerable evidence suggests that many, perhaps most, "retarded" children aren't. Labels should be viewed with caution. In school settings, such labels as "learning disabled," "dyslexic," and "minimally brain damaged" appear to serve another prime purpose: their use instantly and blatantly suggests that the child "has something wrong" and that therefore the teacher, principal, specialists and the entire system should not really be held responsible. To say, "Johnny, in Room 112 in Madison School, under Miss Doe, is not learning to read" is far more uncomfortable than to piously note and record, "Johnny, who lives at 10 Walnut Street, has been diagnosed as dyslexic." The income of many "specialists" also depends heavily on promoting these labels and their use. The "diagnosis" is often treated as though it were medical, but relatively rarely does it reflect a careful examination by a qualified brain-specialist physician, well-experienced in treating children.

CHAPTER 22

1. The key feature of the system that Mann popularized was the graded classroom, on which the entire structure rested and which gave rise to the familiar apparatus of fixed groups, fixed schedules, standardized syllabus and curriculum with subjects and courses, marking, report cards, punishment for control, standardized and graded texts, standardized tests, instruction measured

by elapsed time, rigid and uniform periods, and other regimented operations flatly contrary to recognition of individual differences. Most of this can still be found, very little changed, in almost all our schools.

2. See the Report to the Congress submitted by the U. S. Commissioner of Education, *Education of the Gifted and Talented* (Washington, D. C.: U. S. Government Printing Office, 1972). Findings included that "there is an enormous individual and social cost when talent among the Nation's children and youth goes undiscovered and undeveloped. . . . Gifted and talented children are, in fact, deprived and disadvantaged, and can suffer psychological damage and permanent impairment of their abilities to function well . . . " (p. 68).

3. Recent National Education Association surveys showed 65 percent of elementary and 55 percent of high school teachers favored "judicious use" of corporal punishment. In recent years, thirteen states have passed laws explicitly condoning beating students. A 1971 poll by *Nation's Schools* found 74 percent of respondents stating that corporal punishment was used in their districts. In one large Texas city, over 2,000 uses a month were reported in the 1971–72 school year. See "It's Time to Hang Up the Hickory Stick," *Nation's Schools*, November 1972, pp. 8–9; and Bernard Bard, "The Shocking Facts about Corporal Punishment in the Schools," *Parents' Magazine*, February 1973, p. 44.

4. For a famous investigation of the importance of using speech, see A. R. Luria and F. Yudovich, *Speech and the Development of Mental Processes in the Child* (London and Baltimore: Penguin Papers in Education, Penguin Books, 1971). The study was first published in the U.S.S.R. in 1956.

5. It should not be automatically assumed, of course, that the school in practice wants to facilitate learning by all or most students. The traditional function has been to sort out the sheep and goats. There seems little doubt presently, however, that schools are embarrassed by their inability to prevent massive failure to acquire basic skills and understandings. See Colin Greer, *The Great School Legend* (New York: Basic Books, 1972).

6. See, for example, John C. Flanagan, ed., *The American High School Student* (Pittsburgh: University of Pittsburgh Press, 1964). This is a report on the massive study "Project Talent."

7. See The President's Commission on Law Enforcement and Administration of Justice, *Juvenile Delinquency and Youth Crime* (Washington, D. C.: U. S. Government Printing Office, 1967). The task force reports (p. 223): "Available evidence strongly suggests that delinquent commitments result in part from adverse or negative school experiences of some youth, and, further, that there are fundamental defects within the educational system, especially as it touches lower income youth, that actively contribute to these negative experiences. . . " Other studies support this finding that schools aggressively contribute to crime by what they do to students, as well as by passive failures —what they fail to do for students.

8. *New York Times*, January 16, 1974, special education section, p. 81.

9. See Robert Rosenthal, "The Pygmalion Effect Lives," *Psychology Today*, September 1973, p. 56.

10. Dr. James Coleman, the well-known sociologist and chief author of the "Coleman Report" on equality of education, has written and spoken vigorously

on this point. In a paper, "How Do the Young Become Adults?" he observes: "The student role is not a role of taking action and experiencing consequences. It is not a role in which one learns by hard knocks. It is a relatively passive role, always in preparation for action, but never acting." The young, he adds, "are shielded from responsibility, and they become irresponsible; they are held in a dependent status, and they come to act as dependents; they are kept away from productive work, and they become unproductive." The paper, presented at the American Educational Research Association's 1972 Annual Meeting, was published as *Report Number 130* by the Center for Social Organization of Schools, Johns Hopkins University, Baltimore, Maryland.

11. The visitor to a good open classroom may at first feel that the input level is staggering, because so much is provided by the environment. Visits a week and a month later, however, will reveal that not much in new inputs has been provided. Even when television is utilized, often the same programs are watched week after week. Most of the burden of providing input rests on the teacher, who has much else to do. Quite different arrangements and facilities could, I believe (on the basis of study of new proposals), multiply input perhaps tenfold.

12. For an incisive and widely cited description, see Philip W. Jackson, *Life in Classrooms* (New York: Holt, Rinehart and Winston, 1968), chapter 1. Despite his chilling report, Jackson seems to regard the classroom as an inevitable rather than as an optional structure that should be discarded as soon as possible.

13. John Holt, *Freedom and Beyond* (New York: E. P. Dutton, 1972), p. 243.

14. This figure was widely published in late 1971. For a more recent estimate, see the March 1974 issue of *Esquire*, with the special report "Do Americans Suddenly Hate Kids?" Detailed tables estimate the total cost of raising one child in a well-off urban family as over $31,000 through the first five years, $141,000 through age 17, $189,000 through college (pp. 119–121). Cutting these liberal figures in half results in a figure not far from the earlier estimate.

15. See the series of Gallup Polls, sponsored by CFK, Ltd., a Denver-based (Kettering) foundation, published in *Phi Delta Kappan* from time to time. The poll referred to appeared in September 1962, p. 35.

16. See the report *A Foundation Goes to School*, published by the Ford Foundation, New York, November 1972, summarizing the results of efforts over the period 1960–70; and also the 1972 *Annual Report* of the Charles F. Kettering Foundation, Dayton, Ohio. A Kettering affiliate, Institute for Development of Educational Activities, Inc. (I/D/E/A) has had the most notable success in establishing an actual—rather than lip-service—program of change in over a thousand schools, called Individually Guided Education. The foundation has aided a series of reports, still continuing, including *The Reform of Secondary Education* (New York: McGraw-Hill, 1973), issued by The National Commission on the Reform of Secondary Education, B. Frank Brown, chairman. On the federal front, a large and heavily negative literature exists on the impact of many expensive programs attempted.

17. Christopher Jencks, et al., *Inequality* (New York: Basic Books, 1972), p. 95.

18. Donald Snygg, "A Cognitive Field Theory of Learning," in *Learning*

and Mental Health in the School, 1966 Yearbook of the Association for Supervision and Curriculum Development (Washington, D. C.: National Education Association, 1966), p. 77.

CHAPTER 23

1. See Amitai Etzioni, "Human Beings Are Not Very Easy to Change After All," *Saturday Review*, June 3, 1972, for a perceptive (but nonbrain) discussion by the distinguished Columbia University professor of sociology. He observes that "one of the few effective and efficient ways in which people can be basically remade lies in a total and voluntary reconstruction of their social environment" (p. 47), as when students enter a commune or foreign Jews join an Israeli kibbutz. In such instances, Proster Theory suggests, the biases would be sweepingly altered, permitting much fresh selection of programs, including some newly learned.

CHAPTER 24

1. John E. Pfeiffer, *The Emergence of Man* (New York: Harper & Row, 1969), p. 391.
2. See D. O. Hebb, *Textbook of Psychology*, pp. 214–15. Hebb suggests that our organized social patterns help adults to avoid emotional stimulation, and that we build "cocoons" as further protection.

SUGGESTIONS FOR
FURTHER READING

The selections that follow reflect a personal viewpoint and effort to offer a variety of approaches. The publication dates are of interest: the last half-dozen years have enormously increased the number of nontechnical works of merit, although comprehensive and integrated theory still has been relatively little explored.

Asimov, Isaac. *The Human Brain*. New York: New American Library, 1965. The prolific Dr. Asimov is always clear and informative. A useful general discussion, with attention to hormones.

Beadle, Muriel. *A Child's Mind*. Garden City, N.Y.: Doubleday, Anchor Books, 1971. Focusing on the first five years of life, the book gives much information about newer psychology, with notable clarity.

Calder, Nigel. *The Mind of Man*. New York: Viking Press, 1971. An absorbing account of various aspects of brain research, readable and with many helpful illustrations.

Fink, Donald G. *Computers and the Human Mind*. Garden City, N.Y.: Doubleday, Anchor Books, 1966. An introduction to computers from a human viewpoint, explaining functions, logic, mechanisms, and mathematics.

Gregory, R. L. *Eye and Brain*. 2d ed. New York: McGraw-Hill, 1972. Written for the lay reader with some scientific interests, this survey of "the psychology of seeing" is both fascinating and informative.

Hart, Leslie A. *The Classroom Disaster*. New York: Teachers College Press, 1969. One of the few critical studies of the effects of schools' organization on what they achieve, the book offers some sharp insights into school realities and alternative approaches.

Hebb, D. O. *Textbook of Psychology*. 3d ed. Philadelphia: W. B. Saunders, 1972. A model of a modern, up-to-date text, the work is well worth reading both for content and for the overview it gives.

Hill, Winfred F. *Learning*. Scranton, Pa.: Chandler, 1971. An educator offers a survey of learning psychologies, with some thoughts on the need for a comprehensive theory.

Luria, A. R. *The Working Brain*. New York: Basic Books, 1974. The great Soviet neuropsychologist explains the brain's organization. Though scholarly and technical, the book is not difficult to read.

Mead, Margaret. *Culture and Commitment*. Garden City, N. Y.: Doubleday, Natural History Press, 1970. A discussion of the generation gap and of change in society, this short book holds much significance for all investigating brain-based approaches.

Nathan, Peter. *The Nervous System.* Philadelphia: J. B. Lippincott, 1969. A research neurologist, writing informally and in a highly readable style, gives one of the best introductions for the layman.

Oatley, Keith. *Brain Mechanisms and Mind.* New York: E. P. Dutton, 1972. The English author provides a huge amount of information engagingly, utilizing many pictures and diagrams.

Pfeiffer, John E. *The Emergence of Man.* New York: Harper & Row, 1969. Authoritative and free of technical jargon, this is an outstanding account of the last 25 million years of man's evolution.

Physiological Psychology. San Francisco: W. H. Freeman, 1971. This collection of reprinted articles from *Scientific American* contains a wealth of material on human evolution and behavior and on the brain and its functions.

Pribram, Karl H. *Languages of the Brain.* Englewood Cliffs, N. J.: Prentice-Hall, 1971. For the lay reader, this important work varies widely in readability and technical level. Neuropsychological in approach, it stresses a unified view of the brain's functions.

Rose, Steven. *The Conscious Brain.* New York, Alfred A. Knopf, 1973. This English researcher explains many aspects of origin, organization, and operation on a quite technical level but holds to plain language, often quite informal. Many diagrams help.

Smith, C. U. M. *The Brain.* New York: G. P. Putnam's Sons, 1970. Written lucidly on a technical level, this major, detailed work is best suited to the reader with considerable scientific background. It provides some excellent material on evolution of the brain.

Tiger, Lionel and Fox, Robin. *The Imperial Animal.* New York: Holt, Rinehart and Winston, 1971, Two anthropologists and ethologists explore aspects of human origin and behavior, provocatively, with emphasis on evolution, brain, and learning.

Toffler, Alvin. *Future Shock.* New York: Random House, 1970. This highly popular book, which has had much impact, details our lack of orientation toward the future and surveys the flood of changes we must cope with—areas which invite the application of Proster Theory, as it applies to effecting change.

Travers, Robert M. W. *Man's Information System.* Scranton, Pa.: Chandler, 1970. Addressed to educational technologists, this work focuses closely on perception, information-processing, and a variety of theories.

Wooldridge, Dean E. *The Machinery of the Brain.* New York: McGraw-Hill, 1963. Written by a noted industrial research and development scientist, the book reflects an engineering and computer orientation. It presents stimulating and incisive concepts, and much highly interesting and important material.

INDEX